Choices
In Matters of Life and Death

Judie Brown
with Paul Brown

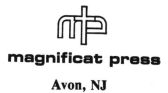

magnificat press

Avon, NJ

Choices
©1987 American Life League
All rights reserved
Printed in the United States of America

ISBN: 0-940543-00-1
Library of Congress catalog card number:
87-060427

Magnificat Press
Avon, NJ 07717

Dedication

To Hugh, Cathy and Christy. May the Lord always protect you and keep you strong. Without you, we might never have known the reality of fighting to make this world a better place for children.

Contents

Part I:
Questions and Answers With Judie Brown

1	In the Beginning—The Origin of Life	1
2	Abortion and Birth Control	11
3	The Complications of Abortion	23
4	How Abortion Became Popular	37
5	How Abortion Became Legal	51
6	The Abortion Industry	63
7	The Mentality of Death	71
8	The Vocabulary of Death	81
9	The Church and Abortion	99
10	Hard Cases	111
11	Tying It All Together	129

Part II:
Questions and Answers With Paul Brown

12	Politics and the Press	139

Appendix A: American Life League 159
Appendix B: Love Is Out, Sin Is In! 163
Notes 169
Index 173

Part I

Questions and Answers
With
Judie Brown

President and Founder of
American Life League

Chapter 1

In the Beginning
The Origin of Life

An argument has been going on for years: What is abortion? And what happens to the baby during an abortion? I think what people really want to know is this: What is life? What is it all about?

Life is a continuum, and each human being is a unique part of this cycle. Life passes on from one person to the next and from one generation to the next. The human race continues because it takes a human sperm and a human egg to create a brand-new human life. If the human egg and the human sperm were not themselves alive, then certainly the product of the union would not be human or very much alive.

Therefore there's no such thing as a "potential" human being. I have the potential to have a baby, but once I actually become pregnant, the baby is real and in existence. There is no such thing as a potential human being in the womb. Each individual life begins at conception, the union of the sperm and egg. Rather than saying that a pregnant woman is going to have a baby, it's really correct to say that she already has a baby.

Once the sperm and the egg unite, what happens? How does the baby grow during the nine months in the womb?

I am going to answer that by quoting from *How Babies Grow*[1]:

Conception (Fertilization): The moment of conception is the beginning of a new human being. The whole genetic information necessary to build our body and our brain is present at this moment. Nothing will be added to this unique individual from the moment of conception except food and nourishment.

First Month: In the next four weeks, this tiny yet distinct embryo which has implanted itself on the uterine wall will be developing its own eyes, spinal cord, nervous system, liver and stomach. At four weeks, the primitive heart, which began beating on the 18th day, is now pumping confidently.

Six Weeks: The baby, a plump little being over a half-inch long with short arms and legs, floats in her amniotic sac, well moored by the umbilical cord. Though she weighs only 1/30 of an ounce, she has all the internal organs of an adult, in various stages of development.

Two months: At eight weeks, she is just over an inch long and everything is present that is found in a full-term baby. This "little one" (the Latin translation is "fetus") must grow. Her hands will soon begin to grip, her feet will try their first gentle kicks and she is able to feel pain.

Three months: The little person floating buoyantly in the amniotic fluid is now more than 2½ inches long. She can make a tiny fist, get hiccups, wake and sleep.

Four Months: The fourth month is marked by rapid growth. If the growth were to continue at this rate throughout the entire pregnancy, the baby would weigh 14 tons at birth. Now external events—especially touch and noise—will reach the baby and provoke reaction.

Five Months: At 20 weeks, she curls as her mother moves, and stretches when her mother rests. She can make an impressively hard fist, and her punches and kicks are felt plainly by her mother. Some preborn children are calm in the womb and others are more active. In this way, she shows her personality.

Seven Months: From the seventh month until term she increases in length from 13 to 20 inches and nearly triples in weight. She experiences the four senses of vision, hearing, taste and touch. This little person now has only to await the miracle of birth.

There you have the history of the first nine months in the life of a brand-new human being. And, as you can plainly see, since all of this material is factual and can be verified in biology textbooks, there can be no question that the brand-new human being exists from the very moment fertilization occurs.

How would you characterize this development of the preborn child?

The beginning of a brand-new human life is nothing less than a miracle because the brand-new human person who exists at the moment of fertilization will never again be created. Each person is unique and distinctly different from the next person, and that unique life begins at the moment when life is in fact created in the womb of a mother, at the moment of fertilization.

Doesn't the Bible have something to say about that?

Yes, the book of Jeremiah tells us that before we were created in the womb, God knew us. He had counted the hairs on our heads and He knew us before fertilization ever occurred, because in God's master plan He knows each and every human being who ever was or ever will be. That reveals the most horrifying aspect of abortion: every abortion eliminates a unique, unrepeatable human person. How many Mother Teresas and Ronald Reagans have been murdered in the womb since 1973?

How many future generations?

That's right.

Is the right to life based exclusively on religious beliefs?

Previously you asked me to describe the development of the human person in the womb. If you read that once again you will see that the biological facts cited there reveal clearly that science has established the development of the human person; religion teaches the involvement of God in this creation. Every human being has a God-given right to live. This principle is stated in the Constitution of the United States; it is as basic as the very fact of our existence.

The founders of our country wrote in the Declaration of Independence that we Americans consider this truth self-evident: all people are "endowed by their Creator with certain inalienable rights," in other words, human rights come from God, and this is obvious to everyone. Among these rights, they said, is the right to life.

I would find it impossible to be deeply involved in the pro-life movement if I didn't have religious convictions about when human life begins. If it were not for God and His power, there would be no creation of human life. God tells us in the Bible that man was created in His image and in His likeness. Therefore each time we destroy a brand-new human being through abortion, we are destroying a creation of God.

If I were a secular humanist, and did not believe in God, but only in myself and my own powers, I would certainly not be motivated to work so hard in the pro-life movement to protect these tiny human beings who will never know me in this life nor know the work we have done to protect their right to life.

If we deny rationally or irrationally the existence of God as the creator of all human life, then it is possible for us as a society to treat ourselves and fellow human beings no differently than we treat whales, snail darters and owls. In fact, if whales or snail darters were being annihilated at the same rate as human beings are today in our society, there would be massive outrage.

It is the responsibility of the pro-life movement to see to it that human beings are once again valued at a much higher level than any animal life, for we are in fact so different, unique and miraculous, because we are created in the image and likeness of God, that we human beings should be the top priority of our society, our government, and every activity that goes on in our country and in our world today. Sadly, we are not.

I hear about the "right-to-life" movement, the "anti-abortion movement," the "pro-life movement." What is the difference?

All of these names really describe the same movement—the work of people who believe that every human being has a God-given right to life, and that human rights should be protected by law.

Pro-life efforts often focus on abortion because that is where the most killing occurs in America today, and because it is currently the one method of killing that is completely legal.

"Pro-life" is the best description of the movement as a whole. The pro-life movement is a total approach to protecting human life, which means that not only are we concerned about the preborn child as long as he or she is living within the womb, and concerned about protecting his or her right to exist, but also we are equally concerned about the families involved with this brand-new human being, particularly the mother.

We must be concerned about handicapped newborn infants, whose lives are threatened today not only after birth but in many cases before birth. We certainly have to be concerned about the elderly whose lives are in jeopardy in the 1980's as never before. Public discussion in our society about the cost of medical care for the elderly and the possibility of having the elderly sign living wills so they can "be put out of their misery" causes pro-life people immense concern. We are totally pro-life. We do not abandon the new child nor do we abandon his or her parents after birth has occurred. Our experience has taught us that we cannot separate abortion from the rest of the life process. The apathy over the more than twenty million abortions that have occurred in our country has given some people the audacity to discuss killing handicapped newborn infants and to discuss whether or not certain members of our human race have no right to continue their existence simply because they happen to be old and sick.

If you protect life at its beginning you must protect life all the way through to its natural end?

The pro-life movement has a moral obligation. We cannot just defend preborn children if we have no intention of defending all innocent human beings and seeing that all innocent human persons are protected. We are constantly being accused of only worrying about children as long as they reside in the womb, but that is a false accusation and one that we have worked very hard to overcome.

On the other hand, a lot of pro-life work has been devoted to legislative and/or political solutions, sometimes ignoring the fact that to this day there are millions of Americans who cannot defend these children who reside in the womb simply because they still do not even know that since January 22, 1973, it has been legal to kill a baby up until the moment of birth.

The legislative and political goals established by the pro-life movement will only succeed when

the majority of Americans articulate their concern
for these babies by supporting, in every way, the
rights of all innocent human beings to live under the
protection of the Constitution.

Chapter 2

Abortion and Birth Control

What is birth control?

Birth control is any method of artificially limiting the number of births. The term "birth control" has nothing to do with the birth of children or the question of self-control. In its various forms, birth control is a part of government programs in many countries around the world to limit population size or to reduce the birth rate among the poor and minorities. Birth control is used by married couples to limit the size of their families. It is often used by single people so they can engage in promiscuous sex without "control" and without a "birth" occurring. However, no method of birth control, not even abortion, is 100 percent effective. Live births often result.

Isn't contraception another word for birth control?

Contraception means the action of a given chemical or device to prohibit fertilization by preventing the sperm from joining with the egg. However, since the promoters of contraceptives are also the promoters of abortion on demand, birth control better describes not only the devices and chemicals in question, but the very philosophy of those promoting it.

Is there a difference between the various forms of birth control (contraceptives)?

A birth control method prevents pregnancy, or at least is supposed to. Condoms and spermicidal sponges are designed to kill the sperm or prevent it from reaching the egg, thereby not allowing fertilization to take place.

However, certain forms of birth control actually work in such a way that they terminate the lives of brand-new human beings. The intrauterine device and the birth control pill in all of its forms, including the new drug RU 486, work to destroy brand-new human life.[2]

How can a birth control method interfere with sperm and egg once they are united? Doesn't the new life just start growing? What happens?

The human sperm and the human egg unite in the fallopian tube to create a brand-new human being. Textbooks call this a zygote.

This new human being travels down the fallopian tube and into the uterus. The trip takes about seven to nine days. When this new human being arrives at the wall of the uterus, he or she has to implant in (attach to) the wall of the uterus to continue to grow and acquire nourishment.

The intrauterine device (IUD) works to inflame the wall of the uterus, to aggravate and agitate it so that the brand-new human being is rejected by the uterine wall. Because of the inflammation he or she cannot implant; thus this brand-new human being dies.

The birth control pill, on the other hand, has two major modes of action. It works to thicken cervical mucus (causing temporary sterility), and to pervent the sperm, if it enters the cervix, from uniting with the egg, by altering the hormonal balance of the womb.

The birth control pill can also work to make the uterine lining totally inhospitable to the fertilized egg, thus causing an abortion to occur.[3] Because we cannot know which of these three actions will take place in the womb, we cannot consider the birth control pill to be contraceptive. We never know when it is causing an abortion.

Because society has never really understood the actions of the birth control pill, it will be a simple matter for the medical profession to foist RU 486 on us. This new chemical, also referred to as a "contraceptive," is a pill that will work only as an early abortion. A woman will be told that if she misses her period, she need not worry about a "possible" pregnancy; she need only take this pill and her worries will be over! Another chemical in the ongoing warfare against babies in the womb, RU 486 has not been approved for use in the United States, and we must work to make sure it never is.

Going back to the brand-new baby, you're saying this baby needs food, and, unable to attach himself or herself to the wall of the mother's uterus, the baby draws no nourishment, and dies?

Yes. If a woman delivers a baby at nine months and no one feeds the baby or provides the proper nourishment, the baby will die. There is no better chance of survival for a newborn human being left unattended than for a brand-new human being who cannot draw nourishment from the wall of the uterus after fertilization.

What happens in abortion?

There are five other basic types of abortion in addition to the pill, the IUD and RU 486.[4] All work to kill a baby that is already growing in the mother's womb.

1. D&C or dilatation-and-curettage abortion. This method is most often used in the first thirteen weeks of pregnancy. A tiny hoe-like instrument, a curette, is inserted into the womb through the dilated cervix, its natural gateway. The abortionist then scrapes the wall of the uterus, cutting the baby's body to pieces. It is now used less frequently than suction.

2. Suction abortion. This method is most commonly used for early pregnancies; the principle in this method is the same as in the D&C. In this technique, which was pioneered in communist China, a powerful suction tube is inserted through the cervix into the womb. The body of the developing baby and the placenta (which connects the baby to the wall of the uterus) are torn to pieces and sucked into a jar.

3. Salt poisoning, saline solution or hypernatremic abortion. This method is generally used after thirteen weeks of pregnancy. A long needle is inserted through the mother's abdomen and a strong saline solution is injected into the amniotic fluid surrounding the child. The salt is swallowed and "breathed" and slowly poisons the baby, and burns the skin as well. The mother goes into labor about a day later and expels a dead, grotesque, shriveled baby. Some babies survive the "salting out" and are born alive.

4. Hysterotomy or caesarean section abortion. In this method, used in the last three months of pregnancy, the abortionist opens the womb surgically through the wall of the abdomen. The baby is removed and allowed to die by neglect, or sometimes killed by a direct act, such as drowning.

5. Prostaglandin chemical abortion. This, a new form of abortion, uses chemicals that are developed and sold by the Upjohn Company of Kalamazoo, Michigan. These hormone-like compounds are injected or otherwise applied to the muscle of the uterus, causing it to contract intensely, thereby pushing out the developing baby. Side effects are many and live births have been common. A self-administered tampon for applying the chemicals is being tested. These abortion chemicals are widely used in the second three months of pregnancy.

At what stage of development are most abortions performed?

Most abortions in the United States (over ninety-five percent) are performed between the moment of fertilization and the end of the third month of development.

How many abortions can a woman have?

There are no statistics to show us how many abortions anyone has obtained, although there are individuals who have come into the pro-life movement admitting to as many as five to seven abortions in their past.[5]

How much does an abortion cost?

The abortion cost varies from state to state and it also depends on whether or not the abortionist is receiving federal or state taxpayer support for the abortion. In the state of California, for example, many times a privately obtained abortion during the first three months of pregnancy will cost as little as $150. However, if the death chamber (abortion clinic) has to apply for state aid (taxpayer dollars) for the abortion, the price can escalate to as high as $400 or more.

The abortion industry is a money-making industry. Abortion continues in this country because it is a multi-million-dollar business.

What do they do with the aborted babies?

That depends on where you live and what the practice of the abortionist is. In some cases the babies are ground up in garbage disposals. In some cases the babies are burned in incinerators. In some cases the babies are stored in garbage bags and taken out to ordinary dumpsters every day when business is complete. We suspect that much of the tissue from aborted children is sold to chemical firms and research firms. An ongoing research project of American Life League is seeking to discover exactly what does happen to aborted babies after they are killed.

Are the babies buried?

No, these children are never buried by the abortionist, although there have been instances where pro-life groups have gone to court and asked for the right to bury these babies' bodies. It is extremely infrequent that a court will allow such burials to take place. What usually happens is that memorial services are held in hundreds of areas around the country to remember these dead children. However, the actual burial of their bodies does not take place in most instances.

Are abortions ever done on fully developed babies?

Of course they are, because abortion is legal in our country up until the moment before birth.

Why do people seek abortion?

The most reasonable response to this question is that after so many years and so many millions of killings, our country has become desensitized to these little children and their right to experience life. I think that many women are forced into the abortion decision by the selfish attitude of those around them, and in countless cases by their own selfishness.

We live in an extremely self-centered society. It is difficult for people to reach out and care enough about their fellow human beings to make personal sacrifices. Until the pro-life movement has taught this country how to hold out its hands to these children and their mothers rather than advising mothers to kill their children, we will not be able to stop the millions of abortions occurring here.

It seems that pro-life people are attempting to stop abortion only through the legislative-political process. Aren't there other ways?

There are many other ways to stop abortion in America. The American society must be converted to believe in the sanctity of each and every human life regardless of its place of residence, its infirmity or its age. Until America believes in the inviolability of human life at every stage of growth, abortion in America will not end.

If abortion is legally banned, how could the abortionists and those seeking abortions be stopped? How would these laws be implemented?

First of all, if abortion were outlawed in America the number of abortions sought or performed would decrease dramatically at once. One of the reasons that abortion is so popular in our nation today is that it is legal and sanctioned by the United States government.

Let us say that abortion were illegal and the laws were upheld by the courts. At that point society would automatically reexamine its position. Of course the hard-core abortion advocates in our country would continue to pursue a woman's ability to kill her baby. But if abortion were illegal in America, few women would break the law to end their pregnancies.

Also our nation would reexamine its entire sexual morality or lack of it. Women and men alike would become far more conscious of the true value of sexual union within marriage as opposed to promiscuous sexual acts outside marriage, particularly for those under the age of eighteen.

I think that the effects of making abortion illegal in America would be far more dramatic than we can imagine. I do not feel, however, that any law should be passed that would put a woman in jail for having undergone an illegal abortion. We must condemn the sin but attempt in every way possible never to condemn the sinner.

On the other hand, the abortionist, who stands to make a tremendous amount of money because of his surgical ability, is the one who should be fined and sentenced should he continue to kill preborn children once the killing is illegal.

Chapter 3

The Complications of Abortion

Judie, we are always hearing about how many women died from illegal abortion—killed with coat hangers and that sort of thing. Aren't abortions performed in clinics or hospitals safe for the women having them? It's a shame that so many babies are killed, but if women are going to have abortions anyway, shouldn't they be safe?

First of all, deaths from illegal abortions had declined rather significantly as early as three to five years before abortion became legal in the United States. The advent of antibiotics contributed a great deal toward lowering the death rate; better treatment was available for women who had suffered at the hands of abortionists.[6] Those who say that more women would die from abortion if it were once again illegal in America are simply using a scare tactic to coerce the public into accepting their pro-death philosophy. Too many women are dying from legal abortions. Women are simply victims of the multi-million-dollar baby-killing business.

Abortion has a traumatic effect on women—not only in a physical way, but in a psychological way as well. Because over seventy percent of the abortions in this country are performed on unmarried young women, the age group of women that has been aborting its children for the last thirteen years has not lived long enough yet for anyone to know exactly how extensive the damage is.

The abortion performed on the immature womb of a teenager may affect her for the rest of her life. If you become pregnant, for example, when you are fourteen years of age, your womb is still developing. The instruments used to take the life of the child living within you can do vast damage to your womb, creating a situation where you may never be able to carry a baby to term. So abortion in America is killing all of these children and ravaging the wombs of women, and we have no idea exactly how much damage has been done.

So if I abort my first baby, I may not be able to bear other children? What else can go wrong?

A woman can be injured, and she can bleed to

death. Here is a list of the 162 most common complications of abortion, excerpted from an excellent book on the subject: *Every Woman Has a Right to Know the Dangers of Legal Abortion* by Ann Saltenberger.[7] It provides over 200 pages of medically documented information. Jose Espinosa, M.D., Herbert Ratner, M.D., and other well-known physicians commend this book to the attention of women. Women who receive "counseling" from Planned Parenthood, women's "health" centers or abortion referral agencies are usually under the impression that they are receiving adequate information. In fact they are not being fully informed of the traumatic side effects of abortion.

The most common *known* complications of abortion:

   Early

abdominal cramps
abdominal surgery
abortion of only one twin
adherent placenta
allergic reaction
amnesia
anemia
anesthetic complications
anuria
aspiration pneumonia

bacterial invasion of the urinary system
birth of a living child during the abortion
bladder damage
blood pressure decrease
blood transfusions
bowel may be sucked out
bowel obstruction
breast engorgement
burns
cerebral edema or damage
cervical detachment
cervical laceration
cervicovaginal fistula
coagulopathy
coma
convulsions
cornual contraction ring with retained placenta
disseminated intravascular coagulation
drug reaction
ectopic pregnancy
electroencephalographic changes
embolism
erythema nodosum
extraperitoneal bleeding
failed abortion
fever
general complications
genital tract infection

headache
hemorrhage
hepatitis
incomplete abortion
incomplete separation of the placenta
infection
injection of salt into a vein
injury to the intestines
intraabdominal uterine rupture
intrauterine loss of the curette tip
isoimmunization
Karman cannula complications
kidney damage and loss
loss of sleep
metabolic complications
milk secretion
multiple organ removal
myocardial infarction
myometrical necrosis
pain
paracervical block reactions
paralytic ileus
particular problems of prostaglandins
pelvic infection
perforation of the bladder
perforation of the bowel
peritonitis
permanent brain damage

pleural effusion
pneumonia
postabortal syndrome (PAS)
posterior cervical rupture
pulmonary complications
pulmonary embolism
pyrexia
renal failure
respiratory infection
retained placenta
retained tissue
rupture of the cervix
rupture of the uterus
salt poisoning
salpingitis
septic incomplete abortion
septicemia
severe reaction to prostaglandin
small bowel obstruction
spleen removal
sterility
suicide
synechia
thromboembolism
thrombophlebitis
torn intestines
transplacental hemorrhage
trauma to the reproductive tract

unintended minor surgery
unnecessary surgery
ureterouterine fistula
urinary tract infections
uterine agony
vomiting
water intoxication
wound dehiscence
wound infection

Late

amenorrhea
birth of a living child
cervical canal diameter increase
cervical incompetence
cervical pregnancy
complicated labors
damage to the myometrium
danger to a later pregnancy
delayed abortion
disruption or infection of wound
dysmenorrhea
ectopic pregnancy
endometriosis
endometritis
fallopian tube damage
frigidity
general bad effects
gross irregularity of menstrual period

implantation of fetal remnants
incapacity
infection
infertility
late termination of pregnancy
miscarriage
ossification in the endometrium
pelvic infection
persistent bleeding
pelvic inflammatory disease
placenta previa
pregnancy potential increase
prolonged hospitalization
prolonged labors
recurrent pregnancy
reduced reproductive capacity
sterility
traumatic intrauterine adhesions

Complications to other children

battering
congenital handicap
damage
developmental problems
death before birth
generally poorer Apgar scores
late spontaneous abortion
low birthweight
perinatal mortality—fifty percent increase

placenta previa
premature labor and delivery
psychiatric problems
risk of central nervous system damage
Rh blood disease
Psychological complications
anguish
depression
grief
numbness
regret
shock
trauma
anxiety
family feticidal syndrome

And the government does nothing about that? It seems to me that the government encourages abortion; don't they require that women be told the truth?

Legally, the physician is not required to inform the woman with regard to the development of her preborn child. Further, he is not required to provide her with, at the very least, the listing of complications which you have just read. The United States Supreme Court ruled, in 1976, 1981, and again in 1986 that providing certain facts to the

pregnant mother considering an abortion is simply
an undue burden upon her. Politicians, in turn, no
matter what their positions may be with the government, are easily "off the hook" with regard to
demanding that this information be made known
simply because they can turn to the Supreme Court
and point out that, after all, "it is the law of the
land" and that the government should not interfere
in medical practice.[8]

Though this may sound like bad governing to
you, the fact of the matter is that ambivalence has
so penetrated our nation's law-making bodies that
scarcely a word is uttered, except by a valiant few,
with regard to the woman's right to know. And in
addition, the many so-called "women's rights"
groups in our nation deny the existence of these
realities while continuing to promote the killing of
preborn babies, the ravaging of wombs, the anni-
hilation, if you will, of their own future members.
"Women's rights" stop short of protecting women
from the physically and psychologically devastating
after-effects of abortion.

*Isn't having an abortion a lot safer than a nor-
mal delivery of a live baby?*

No. In the first place, abortion is nearly 100
percent fatal for the baby. Even among babies born

alive accidentally, crying and kicking, only a very few have been allowed to live.

In the second place, the supposed safety of abortion for the mother has been greatly overstated.[9] The women physically or psychologically injured by abortion often don't know where to turn with their problems, and consequently the problems may not be reported. Most women who have abortions are required by the abortionists to sign a waiver exempting the abortionists from responsibility for complications.

The psychological effects of abortion compared to childbirth are particularly more severe. There aren't many women suffering psychological trauma from giving birth to their children. As the Bible says, a mother is so filled with joy over her new baby that she forgets the pain (John 16:21). On the other hand, a study[10] by Dr. Anne Speckhard of the University of Minnesota found that more than half of the women who have had abortions suffered from nightmares and flashbacks related to their abortion experiences. Nearly one in four experienced hallucinations; thirty-five percent believed their dead baby returned to visit them in dreams or visions.

What about the long-term psychological problems you mentioned—do women's health centers and Planned Parenthood offer help to deal with those? Where can a woman get help?

In general, the abortion industry does not care to acknowledge the numerous health problems due to abortion. Feminists (at least those who preach a woman's "right" to abortion; not all do) tend to view women who claim injury due to abortions as traitors to the women's movement.

However, there are many avenues of help for women who have experienced psychological problems from aborting their children.[11] Especially helpful are those groups composed of women who have themselves suffered from abortion; they exist in every state.[12]

We in the pro-life movement are concerned with every life, and with the quality of every life. We not only want to see every innocent human life protected; we want also to help the mothers and their children. Birthright, for example, not only defends the right to life; in fact, most of their efforts are given in support of mothers who need help, providing them with baby clothes, furniture, even places to live if possible.

We genuinely care about women and children. Most of the work of the pro-life organizations I mentioned is done by unpaid volunteers; the organizations are supported solely by private donations.

Don't they receive government support? Helping mothers and their babies sounds like a worthy social program.

No, they don't want any money from the government. Until recently, in order to receive taxpayer support, a group had to be willing to counsel for abortion. Because pro-life post-abortion counseling groups and others are unwilling to recommend the killing of preborn children as a solution to any problem, they simply have not been eligible for the millions of taxpayer dollars that go only to those groups willing to support the killing.

Chapter 4

How Abortion Became Popular

Judie, if scientists agree that human life begins at conception, and if abortion has so many dangers and complications for the mother, how did it become so popular? It doesn't seem to me that women just make up their minds and run down to have an abortion. How did we in the United States get to this point where we are killing 1.6 million children per year? How did it happen?

You have to create an attitude, in society, that abortion is an acceptable thing.

It all started back in 1915 when Margaret Sanger,[13] who ultimately became the founder of Planned Parenthood Federation of America, began extolling the virtues of sterile sexual relationships between poor husbands and wives. She said that her goal was to create a situation whereby poverty-stricken couples would not have one child after another so quickly that many women would die in childbirth, because they were not prepared physically to have so many children so close together.

But while that was the public attitude of Margaret Sanger, her private attitude was anti-black, anti- any minority, and she used terms such as "human weeds" to describe the children of the very people she publicly said she was trying to help.

If I had to use a word to describe Margaret Sanger and all of those people who traveled in her circles, I would call them "eugenicists." Eugenics is the science of purifying a race. What Adolf Hitler did in Germany was in fact advocated by Margaret Sanger in America.

You make it sound like Margaret Sanger was something of a racist. I've seen films that show her as a heroine of the feminist movement.

Her philosophy, which was and still is at the foundation of Planned Parenthood's philosophy, involved limiting births among "undesirables." One of her favorite sayings was "More children from the fit; less from the unfit." Her plans to force sterilization and abortion on the "weak-minded" poor would not have been easy to implement in a democratic society, however. The average American would have recoiled at her organization's desire to eliminate the poor and the weak.

So did Planned Parenthood change its philosophy?

Not really. Even today Planned Parenthood supports forced abortion where it is politically feasible, as in China. They have not changed their philosophy—they have simply popularized public acceptance of birth control and abortion, providing abortions, and breaking down traditional morality by attacking parents, the family and the churches.

I don't agree with forcing women to abort their babies, but isn't some population control necessary? Aren't we in danger of overpopulation?

No, we are in danger from self-centered materialism, from worship of convenience. It is true, there is much human suffering from famine and poverty. But it's not true that we must blame the poor for having too many children. It's much harder to address the real reasons for poverty and famine, reasons such as exploitation and stone-age farming. The fact is that we as a human family are not living up to our responsibilities; we are socially in tune with our own comfort, not the self-sacrifice required of each of us if we are to truly resolve poverty by giving of our own prosperity.

Let's look a little closer at the myth of over-population, because it has been used to justify all kinds of evil.

The population control movement actually started in the late 1700's with the writings of Thomas Malthus, who declared that it was necessary to control the number of people on the earth. Malthus preached that by the early 1900's the world would be so populated that there wouldn't be enough room for all of us. Even at that early date in our history, birth control methods were being discussed, and among them was abortion.

It is unfortunate that those who promote abortion tell us repeatedly that they do not believe in abortion as a form of birth control, because their own leaders in the past definitely viewed it that way.

Alan Guttmacher's early research concluded that at conception a new life begins, a composite of all the hereditary material of father and mother. His book *Life in the Making* (1933) set forth his evidence that a complete human being exists from the moment of conception.

In the 1960's, however, as the president of Planned Parenthood, he was arguing for legal abortions as a means of birth control. By this time he had stopped talking about the humanity of the unborn child.

The overpopulation myth was also fueled more recently by Hugh Moore and Paul Ehrlich.[14]

Hugh Moore, the Dixie Cup millionaire, in the late 1960's, was promoting his idea that the world was in a crisis of overpopulation, which he blamed on the Roman Catholic Church. He purchased full-page ads in newspapers all across America to preach his message, trying to mold public opinion, and to some extent he succeeded. He warned people that the Roman Catholic Church wanted to control America, and that if it did, there would be millions and millions of people falling off the earth.

He engaged a research scientist by the name of Paul Ehrlich to write a book called *The Population Bomb*. Paul Ehrlich's book was released as Hugh Moore's full-page ads began to appear in 1968. The public read the ads and felt that they were accurate, and began to believe that there were too many people in the world and that something had to be done.

In effect, public opinion was molded by the rich. Margaret Sanger's Planned Parenthood was also sponsored by a rich man. Sanger left her first husband and her children and eventually wound up divorcing her husband. Noah Slee, her second husband, was heir to the Three-in-One Oil fortune. He provided millions of dollars to fund her and her activities, especially her major interest: controlling the children of minorities and children of the poor.

The people who changed public opinion were what the common man would view as elitists, people who wanted more of everything for themselves and less for those of the lower classes.

These merchants of death got started with money from Three-in-One Oil, from the Ford Foundation, the Rockefellers, General Motors and others.

With the growing public sentiment in favor of population control, eventually the federal and state governments got involved with funding family-planning programs. Today abortion propagandists, including Planned Parenthood, receive millions in federal funds (your tax dollars) in addition to foundation and corporate support.

Well, family planning isn't all bad, is it? Don't just about all the Christian churches accept family planning?

Prior to 1930, no church body in the world accepted artificial birth control. They went to the Bible and the teaching of the Old Testament in particular to support their opposition.

In 1930 at the Lambeth Conference in England, the Anglican church determined that there were some hardship cases where couples could use artificial birth control. Once birth control was accepted by this very influential church, the Anglican church, even for just a few cases, it made an opening for broad changes. The proponents of abortion and sexual freedom, sexual expression, promiscuity, pornography and divorce hammered away at the opening.[15]

Today in our country, there are countless numbers of Christians and Jews who don't even remember their own history. What is accepted by them today as common practice was known up until 1930 to be a terrible sin against the law of God.

When the exception for hard cases occurred, allowing birth control, the floodgates for promiscuity were opened.

Churches, no matter what church it is, are supposed to represent the biblical teachings. But church leaders themselves began in the thirties to create exceptions to the teachings of their own churches. As many churches gave in on birth control, even on abortion, they made it easy for entire governments all around the world to make exceptions and change the laws that protected human life. And governments are denying the rights of innocent human beings today because the churches in the thirties made exceptions to Biblical teachings.

Where else did support for abortion and birth control come from? To get to where we are today must have take more than compromise on the part of the churches.

The compromise on the part of the churches coincided with a movement in our country to divorce government from moral principles as embodied in God's laws. This effort to separate the nation's laws from the religious principles on which the United States was founded was destined to create chaos.

John Dewey, for instance, had a tremendous influence on public education in the United States. He was a philosopher and educator, and he was part of this movement to remove religious influence from government, and particularly from education. Like the proponents of birth control, those who worked to get God out of government and education claimed to be working for freedom. But neither group, although they pretended to be democratic, really represented the thoughts or wishes of the American people. This philosophy of man as God was pushed by an elite group of people who wanted to change, and did change, the direction of this country. They worked to take away the human right to life, to take away religious freedom, to take away morality—by calling each an infringement of the individual's right to privacy.

Margaret Sanger presented motherhood as

slavery and promiscuity as freedom. Today we have people like Gloria Steinem and Betty Friedan calling Christianity a mental illness, labelling religious instruction an abridgement of children's rights, and calling atheism freedom.

So you're saying that a basic reversal in values has been taking place, with one thing leading to another.

The cry for birth control and population control led eventually to promiscuity, our present high divorce rate, abortion on demand.

Those who demanded unlimited abortion began their crusade by concentrating on the hard cases. This led to the 1973 Supreme Court decision allowing abortion in virtually any case.

Once the government began to compromise on the right to life, it became very difficult to stop with just abortion. Especially with court cases concerning human life, one decision becomes a precedent for the next, a stepping stone to take the right to life away from one more person or class of persons.

On the other hand, advances in medicine and science are making it harder to deny the evidence that each unique, sacred human life begins at conception (fertilization).

This is one reason we are so anxious to see the

Supreme Court review its decision; although there
are many moral questions about *in vitro* fertilization, one thing is crystal clear, and that is that
medicine today, beyond a shadow of a doubt,
recognizes that life begins at fertilization.

If biological scientists were to go before the
Supreme Court today with Louise Brown, the very
first *in vitro* baby in England, the Court would be
hard-pressed to deny the obvious. The Court would
be required once and for all either to say that they
are legalizing the killing of human beings in
America or, as we hope, to reverse themselves and
say that brand-new human beings exist in the
wombs of mothers from the moment of fertilization and therefore are deserving of equal protection
under the law.

What do you mean by in vitro *fertilization?*

In vitro fertilization is a scientific procedure
which allows an infertile woman to possibly have a
child. The egg is taken from her fallopian tube and
is united with her husband's sperm in a petri
dish—a glass laboratory dish. (*In vitro* means "in
glass.") The resultant fertilized egg is then placed in
her womb so that a pregnancy, which has already
begun in the petri dish, can continue within a womb
otherwise thought to be sterile.[16]

With *in vitro* fertilization, you have the developing baby living, initially, outside the mother. It's hard to deny that you have an independent person.

Now, in Germany during the Second World War, they declared the Jew a non-person. Isn't that basically what the Supreme Court has done to the preborn child—called him a non-person?

That's right.

So it is easier to kill somebody who is not a human being?

That is why pro-life people repeatedly say that abortion leads to euthanasia, and to the termination of newborn infants' lives if they happen to be handicapped.

The goal of abortion proponents, funded by enormous foundations with millions of dollars, is to make it acceptable in our country and around the world to eliminate human beings regardless of where they live—whether they live in the womb or in the rest home.

But aren't Americans today very concerned about life? Look at the environmental movement.

Environmental organizations today have concentrated so heavily on the preservation of certain species of animals that they have degraded man. They have actually come to look upon man as another animal and believe the population explosion myth. They are more concerned with saving animal life such as whales, seals, snail darters, owls and hawks. They are equally concerned about controlling the numbers of human beings who live on the earth because they view human beings, another animal form, as a threat to the animals they claim are "endangered species."

You know, Judie, there is another contradiction in our society, and maybe you can explain it. No matter what political label is applied, when you deal with population, don't you find people on both sides who would like to kill people? Who want fewer people on the earth?

Yes, and I think that is why we try very hard in the pro-life movement to divorce ourselves from political labels. The pro-life philosophy is not shared by many conservatives the same way that it is not shared by many of the ultra-liberals in our society. I believe there are just as many fiscally conservative Republicans who are willing to terminate preborn children's lives—and the lives of anybody else who gets in the way—as there are liberals. Their reasons may be different, but the motives are exactly the same.

In other words, the rich get richer and the poor get off the face of the earth. Is that the basic philosophy?

Oh, that is an excellent description of their philosophy.

Chapter 5

How Abortion Became Legal

Judie, not too long ago, a young woman died having an abortion. Her parents were shocked, and the community was shocked to find that abortion itself was legal through the ninth month of pregnancy. What happened to the laws that existed until 1973? What did the Supreme Court do?

On January 22, 1973, the United States Supreme Court decided (in *Roe v. Wade* and *Doe v. Bolton*) by a 7-to-2 vote that under no circumstances except a very limited one in the last three months of pregnancy could our society prevent a woman from having an abortion. In simpler terms, the Court said that from the moment of fertilization until the actual moment of birth, abortion would be legal in America.

The one restriction the Court put on abortion in its decision was that during the last three months of pregnancy, for the sake of the mother's health alone, abortions had to be performed in a hospital and two physicians had to concur with regard to the need for abortion.

However, we have learned that this is absolutely no restriction when one considers that any explanation on the part of the woman is acceptable to most of the medical profession and therefore abortion is performed for any reason whatsoever throughout the nine months of pregnancy.

I know that after this 1973 decision many attempts were made to have the Supreme Court reverse its decision, and to defend the rights of parents to be involved in their daughters' abortion decisions. What has the Court said about this?

In 1976, the Supreme Court, in *Planned Parenthood v. Danforth*, decided that parents could not be involved in their daughter's decision to abort a child even if their daughter were an unemancipated minor.

What is an unemancipated minor?

An unemancipated minor is a child under the age of eighteen who resides with a parent or legal guardian. An emancipated minor would be one who is married or who has moved away from home on her own. But as long as a child lives at home or with a guardian, that child is considered unemancipated, not free to make decisions on his or her own. A girl cannot, for example, have her ears pierced unless her mother signs an approval slip, but she can kill a baby and her parents have no right to interfere, according to the Supreme Court.

What are the father's rights in an abortion?

None. In 1976, again in *Planned Parenthood v. Danforth*, the Court ruled that, because a mother has her own right to privacy, regardless of who was involved in creating the brand-new human life, the father has no rights.

Since that decision, fathers in many states have tried in vain to stop their wives, or in some cases boyfriends have tried in vain to stop their girlfriends, from aborting their babies, but in case after case the courts have ruled that the woman has her own private right to choose to end the life of her child and the husband or boyfriend has absolutely no rights at all.

Earlier you described how some birth control methods destroy new human life. Did the Court deal with this in its 1973 decision?

Well, if we study the Court's decisions and try to see when the Court began arbitrarily granting the right to kill, we have to go back to 1965 when the last of the so-called Comstock Laws or the old birth control laws in America was overturned by the Supreme Court.

In that decision, *Griswold v. Connecticut*, which I think is the most significant Supreme Court decision ever, the Court created the "right to privacy." There never has been in the U.S. Constitution a right to privacy, but in 1965, to legalize all forms of birth control for married couples, the Court ruled that couples have a "right to privacy" and therefore the state has no compelling interest, even in alerting them to the medical side effects of birth control. This contrived "right to privacy" laid the groundwork for further anti-life actions by the Court.

Justice Stewart agreed that the "right to privacy" was contrived and could not be found in the Constitution. In his dissenting opinion on *Griswold v. Connecticut*, he wrote: "In the course of its opinion the Court refers to no less than six amendments to the Constitution: The First, the Third, the Fourth, the Fifth, the Ninth and the 14th. But the Court does not say which of these amendments, if any, it thinks is infringed by this Connecticut law.

"What provision of the Constitution, then, does make this law invalid? The Court says it is the right of privacy 'created by several fundamental constitutional guarantees.' With all deference, I can find no such general right of privacy in the Bill of Rights, in any other part of the Constitution, or in any case ever before decided by this Court.

"At the oral argument in this case we were told that the Connecticut law does not 'conform to current community standards.' But it is not the function of this Court to decide cases on the basis of community standards. We are here to decide cases 'agreeable to the Constitution and laws of the United States.' "

In 1972, in *Eisenstadt v. Baird*, the Supreme Court again referred to the "right to privacy," ruling that contraceptives may be given to unmarried individuals, concluding that the "equal protection under the law" guaranteed by the Constitution confers the rights of married persons on the unmarried as well.

What the Court did in 1973 was simply to carry forward that right to privacy created in 1965 and legalize the killing of innocent preborn children.

Did they rationalize the decision in 1973 by saying that they had already allowed killing of brand-new human beings through some forms of birth control?

Well, let's get one thing straight, first. The Supreme Court never looked at medical evidence. The Supreme Court set aside all the medical evidence available to it in 1973 and based both of its decisions that year on women's rights.

The Court said that they could not determine when human life begins and shouldn't be asked to do so. They reasoned, falsely, that if theologians, ethicists and misguided physicians could not decide when life begins, then they certainly could not. So in 1973 the Court wouldn't have been concerned about the pill and the IUD terminating new human life because they said they didn't know when human life begins or even if a human being exists in a mother's womb during pregnancy—that's why they weren't concerned that abortion and birth control kill babies.

Our society can put a man on the moon but cannot decide when human life begins?

Yes, and that is only one of the ironies in this matter. If you look at the comments made by abortion proponents you will hear repeatedly that women's rights are of paramount importance and that we, the pro-life movement, have no concern about women's rights.

But, frankly, no one who promotes abortion will detail the complications of abortion, nor display the anguish, the pain, the physical harm that is done to women time and time again in abortion. I think that if we get right down to it, we in the pro-life movement are the only ones working to defend a woman's right to know. We're just not defending her "right" to kill her child.

I seem to recall a recent Supreme Court decision that was somewhat of a victory for life. Could you explain that?

In the Akron decision (*City of Akron v. Akron Center for Reproductive Health*, 1983), the Court did determine that some kinds of further restrictions can be applied to a third-trimester pregnancy. They did approve a limited type of informed consent. But if we look at what actually happened as a result of this case, we can see that their decision actually worked to protect abortion chambers, the places where babies are killed, and not so much to protect women.

The Akron Ordinance required parental notice and consent before an unemancipated minor child could obtain an abortion. The United States

Supreme Court said no to parents, thus saying yes to the abortion chamber's counseling of the young.

The Akron Ordinance required that facts concerning the development of the baby in the womb and the complications of abortion be detailed before a mother made the final decision to terminate the life of her preborn child. The United States Supreme Court said no to information of this nature, thus telling abortion chambers to continue giving only those bits of information that would lead a pregnant woman or a young girl into the decision to take the life of the child within her. Another victory for the abortion chamber.

The Akron Ordinance required that proper burial be given to the dead child after the abortion was complete. The United States Supreme Court said no to this simple request for humane treatment of the corpse, thus enabling the abortion chamber to continue using its incinerators, its garbage dumpsters or its garbage disposals. Another victory for the abortion chamber.

The Akron Ordinance required that women who decide upon an abortion during the fourth month of pregnancy or after be hospitalized before the surgical killing is done. The Supreme Court ruled that this placed a burden on the pregnant mother's ability to obtain an abortion, thus providing the abortion chambers with still another victory.

The Akron Ordinance required that once a woman decided upon an abortion, she should wait twenty-four hours before submitting to this serious surgical procedure. The United States Supreme Court ruled that this waiting period simply increased the financial costs to the pregnant mother because she would have to make two trips to the abortion chamber, thus they ruled out the waiting period.

To summarize the Akron decision, we see clearly that, again in 1983, the Supreme Court acted against the child who resides in the womb, against the pregnant woman, against the parents of unemancipated minor children, and in favor of keeping down the costs of killing and keeping open the doors of the chambers of death, known as abortion clinics.

The Court has done nothing in the last twenty years to protect women, to give them enough information to make an informed decision.

Take the case of a fifteen-year-old girl who finds out that she is pregnant, and she goes to a school counselor rather than to her mother. Because she is so distressed, it is easy to talk her into an abortion if you fail to give her all the facts.

And even after the Akron decision, there is no requirement in our country to tell a pregnant woman exactly how much the baby has developed in her womb. What size is her baby? How much does her baby weigh? None of that is told to a woman contemplating abortion. Abortionists say it would only incite nervous reaction on the part of the pregnant woman.

Do you mean to tell me that a fifteen-year-old child can legally have an abortion without her parents knowing about it?

Oh, yes! In fact, in many high schools in America today there are actually clinics right in the high school. These clinics in schools are called "Comprehensive Health Clinics" but they are really clinics to condone promiscuous sex and abortion. A student can go to the clinic during a lunch hour, make an appointment and be taken to have an abortion. She will be back in class that same day and her parents will never know! (See Appendix B for more on school-based clinics.)

Well, what if something happened to the girl when she had an abortion, and she had complications? Who would be liable for that?

The parents are liable for any complications resulting from an aborton.

That doesn't really seem right. You mean that if a child has an abortion, that's okay, and the parents have no say in it?

That's right.

But if the child has an abortion and becomes ill or dies, or has major medical complications during the abortion, the parents then become liable, after the fact?

Yes, that's right. When the teenager enters the clinic she will be given a form. The form she is asked to sign releases the medical facility from any accountability after the abortion is complete. Parents who have no right to know certainly cannot contact the clinic if a release form is signed.

This then protects the clinic from any ramifications should the girl die, or hemorrhage, or become sterile later in life. She herself would have no recourse if years after her abortion, as a legal adult, she discovered that she was sterile and could never have a child.

Then to sum it up, the Supreme Court has ruled, obviously again and again, that a woman today has a right to privacy. And that her right to privacy prevents anyone from interfering with her decision to have an abortion?

Her decision with her physician. That is correct. That is a private decision.

So her parents are out, husbands are out, everyone else is out?

Right. And especially the baby. The baby is always out.

Chapter 6

The Abortion Industry

Judie, many people today are confused by all the rhetoric. So many people are arguing for "abortion rights." What does the National Organization for Women, for example, have to do with abortion?

In order to be a member of the National Organization for Women, you must accept their principle that a woman has a right to choose to kill her preborn baby. The latest efforts of the National Organization for Women center on harassment of the pro-life service agencies throughout the country, in addition to their continued harassment of pro-life organizations in general. They consistently make fanatical claims to the press.

The president of the National Organization for Women has repeatedly claimed that it is pro-life people who are perpetrating much of the bombing of abortion chambers in America. She has never substantiated her claim but continues to travel around the country, trying to destroy the very character of the pro-life movement itself.

How about the Equal Rights Amendment? Why do pro-life groups oppose that?

Well, the National Organization for Women and all other radical feminist organizations claim that the Equal Rights Amendment itself has absolutely nothing to do with the expansion of abortion on demand. But in federal court cases in Hawaii, Pennsylvania and Massachusetts, to name just three states, the courts have ruled that a woman's right to abortion is guaranteed by state Equal Rights Amendments. Therefore, it is mandatory for those in the pro-life movement to continue to adamantly oppose the Equal Rights Amendment, both state versions and on the national level.

What about ZPG—Zero Population Growth? Are they only for a stable population size or do they actively promote abortion?

All of the organizations that promote a no-growth population, not only for our country but around the world, are equally guilty of promoting abortion on demand as one of the ways to control population size. Zero Population Growth is one of many such organizations that claim to be concerned about the rights of individuals to food, clothing and proper housing, but who are in fact behind the anti-life movement here and around the world.

Is it true that Planned Parenthood makes quite a bit of its money actually performing abortions?

Yes, that is true. In 1985 they performed at least 85,000 abortions in their own death chambers.[17]

Some other groups that have nice-sounding names are also involved, to a degree, in promoting abortion, but many people aren't aware of it.

The March of Dimes consistently presents a public image of being in favor of children and doing everything they possibly can to assist those born with handicaps. But the facts speak for themselves. The March of Dimes is guilty of continuing to fund research studies that claim to show the safety of abortion; at the same time the March of Dimes is deeply involved in such things as promotion of genetic engineering and development of permissive sex instruction courses. Most recently, the March of Dimes is encouraging placement of school-based sex clinics as well.

How about the United Way? Why do pro-life groups object to funding United Way?

The United Way in various parts of the country gives money to organizations such as Planned Parenthood. Recent research by our office has shown that the United Way funds many "service" organizations that promote abortion, refer for abortion, or encourage young women to have abortions.

If I were making a decision about support of groups dealing with genetic defects, I would certainly not support either the United Way or the March of Dimes but would give all of my money to the Michael Fund. The Michael Fund is a pro-life research institute totally dedicated to discovering cures for genetic defects.

How big an industry is abortion in this country?

There are hundreds of millions of dollars involved on a yearly basis. There actually are abortion clinic franchises (chains) throughout the country. There are two chains in existence now. The first is the Feminist Women's Health Center, which has death chambers located in the South and in the Southeast and also in the West. In Dallas, Texas, there is yet another franchise system of death chambers. Businessmen have made large investments in these death chambers and simply lease out the business to various abortion-promoting doctors.

Then there is Dr. Allred in California. He has a series of death chambers which he calls offices but which we know are part of a very large death-promotion business. Dr. Allred is the one who several years ago said that if it were possible for him to do so he would open an abortion chamber at the United States–Mexico border because he felt it was necessary for Mexicans to have abortions any time they were pregnant. He is another one of the racist individuals behind the abortion industry in this country.

Why hasn't big business opposed abortion? Don't they stand to lose money? Don't they realize just how much financial loss they are suffering by reducing the number of babies?

It seems that big business is the last to take a moral stand. I don't think that large corporations have addressed the financial ramifications of over twenty million abortions in this country. I think sometimes that is due to ignorance. At other times it is due to the amount of pressure which abortion proponents put on these firms.

Meanwhile, the pro-life movement exists on so many small donations that it simply has not been possible for us to compete with the abortion industry in manipulating big business. I am hopeful that we will begin to gain influence with them anyway, however, by discussing, for example, how many boxes of Pampers will never be sold because twenty million children have been put to death. But as yet I do not see those discussions taking place.

You mentioned earlier that the Rockefeller and Ford Foundations fund Planned Parenthood and other anti-life groups. How can pro-lifers start to have an impact on some of these foundations and at least get them out of the business of financing abortion around the world?

Our first obstacle to overcome is the ignorance of corporate officials. In two cases, one being the Kellogg Corporation and the other IBM, the pro-life movement was successful in getting each of these corporations through their foundations to deny continued funding for Planned Parenthood. It was an educational process that took many letters from individuals across this country to the presidents of these two corporations.

It is our moral obligation to educate all those

in positions of power so that decisions about charitable gifts are made with all the facts. When they contribute to Planned Parenthood, they sincerely believe they're helping people. We have to convince them that abortion isn't charity.

Chapter 7

The Mentality of Death

Judie, it seems to me that a sort of mentality of death prevails not just for babies in the womb but all the way to the tomb. Socialized killing seems to have become an accepted solution. How has that happened?

Well, our society has lost its will to live. We have committed national suicide. We have taken the lives of over twenty million human beings without paying any attention to the effect the killing has had on our society. Today there are so many elderly and so many more from the baby boom generation who will be elderly that our government and our society as a whole has become concerned about how we are going to deal with the massive numbers of elderly people we will have within the next twenty to forty years.

But at the same time as we have developed this

concern, we have lost our respect for life. And I believe that the generation coming up—one that has lost twenty million to abortion—will one day turn on their very parents, who aborted their siblings, their brothers and sisters. They will terminate their own parents for the very reasons that those parents determined it was right and legal for them to terminate the lives of the preborn. Those who will be making life-and-death choices in the future will have lost brothers and sisters for no reason at all. They will see nothing wrong with taking the life of an elderly or terminally ill relative (through euthanasia).

If a child's parents can kill him, you are saying that when the child grows up, he can also kill the parents. Is that happening today?

Oh, yes, the abortion mentality of death as a solution is certainly spreading.

In Europe there is an organization called Exit, which publishes handbooks on suicide. One of the founders of that organization, Derek Humphry, also founded an organization in Los Angeles called the Hemlock Society.

During the last couple of years that society has reached national attention. Mr. Humphry has published his own handbook on suicide in this country and actually travels around the country and receives national media attention for his advocacy of what he calls assisted suicide, but which many of us would call murder.

Well, if you go walking through the corridors of a nursing home today, you see many elderly people who have lost their so-called quality of life, who aren't really productive members of society any more. It is claimed that these elderly people have become a financial drain on their families. What's wrong with the families letting these persons die?

The family doesn't "let" anyone die. Nature will take its course; an elderly person will ultimately die of natural causes. We have lost our recognition of the fact that perhaps Grandma or Grandpa is incapacitated, but that their wisdom has made a tremendous contribution to our family and to the community.

Now we are ready as a society to take them and throw them away as though they were nothing but human garbage. This is called euthanasia.

But aren't we on the road to euthanasia? It seems to me that with a smaller work force supporting a growing elderly population and with the troubles that Social Security has seen in recent years

and will probably see again—won't these just give
more and more reason to get rid of the elderly? I
don't see much hope for them.

I don't see any hope for the elderly if the abortion mentality in our country continues to grow,
because, again, as a nation, we have lost our will to
live. We have decided that life is cheap and that certain human beings are expendable. We made that
decision in 1973 and today we are killing 4,000
human beings a day without thinking much of it.

Recent court decisions in California, New
Jersey and elsewhere make it very clear that even
giving food and water to an elderly person can be
considered by the courts to be extraordinary means
of treatment. Certain courts in our country have
decided that it is legal to starve a patient to death
simply because the patient is ill or senile or not dead
yet, but "should" be. When the courts begin to
make decisions like that, we are on the road to
death whether we like it or not, and all of us are on
that road.

It seems to me, Judie, that we have let the
government and perhaps the lawmakers take over
the decisions that used to be made by families. We
have forgotten common sense when an elderly per-
son is near death. I don't know if anyone really

believes that we should prolong suffering just to let someone live another day or week or an hour. What do we do about that?

Well, the trouble is that we have legislators fanatically pursuing the fears that many doctors have about being sued for malpractice.

Twenty years ago, or even ten years ago, if a person were on the verge of death, the physician and the family would discuss the condition and would make a determination that certain types of medical treatment, such as an extra machine, were not necessary because there was nothing that anyone could do to bring the person back. Medical professionals used to assist families in determining what kind of ordinary treatment was needed to keep a person comfortable, nourished and as aware as possible of his or her family members, but at the same time recognizing that death was imminent.

Today, on the other hand, quite often no common sense is employed whatsoever. We have situations where a person who may have two or three days to live gets plugged into a multitude of machines to protect the physician, and on the other hand, we have persons who advocate terminating all kinds of treatment including basic antibiotics, food and water in order to hasten death.

So you are saying we should apply common sense, that we should make a person comfortable, but that we should not speed up death?

Yes. We know, for example, that all pain is manageable now and that some forms of drug therapy given to people in indescribable pain will do other damage, but at the same time make them comfortable. That is the kind of treatment that should be given to a dying person.

But until the moment a person is pronounced dead, he is still alive and deserving of every compassionate effort that can be made to protect his life.

But what do you say to the abortionists, the euthanasiasts, the people who bring out these hard and very sad cases? The average person just reading the story in the papers thinks, gee, that sounds reasonable, people who are in comas should be allowed to die. How do we overcome that? How do we answer them in a reasonable way to show that we are perhaps more caring than they are?

By the use of compassion. Our society has lost its compassion and begun to treat the elderly and the extremely ill in the same way that it began to treat pregnant women in the late sixties. Our society has tried to desensitize families, to make them look upon their elderly and their hopelessly ill as strains on the pocketbook rather than as valuable human beings who should be cherished right up to the very end.

It goes back to the loss of respect for life. Our society has equated the value of each and every human being with so many financial and economic terms that we have lost our ability to see each and every human being as uniquely special.

Then a dollar value has been placed on human life, economic value rather than a compassionate value?

Yes, and we can see the dollar value used in regard to birth control for teenagers. Our opponents tell us that for every dollar spent, $1.83 is saved. What that really means is that they are willing to sell sex to teens with "protection" rather than teach them the value of chastity.

We are told that for every abortion performed on a young woman, our society saves a great deal of money in welfare. That is unproven by all of the economic studies that have been done because most young women who have children will be back into the work force or back into school if only society provides a little bit of help.

But our society would rather terminate the

baby and not have to worry about helping the family after birth occurs. And now our society is going to apply the same kind of arguments to the elderly. It is only a matter of time.

It seems to me the proponents of abortion should start worrying about themselves as they approach retirement age.

They won't concern themselves so much with their own ultimate demise because they don't believe in a life hereafter, they don't believe in accountability to God, they think they have absolutely nothing to lose.

If you listen to some of them, especially those who have terminated members of their own families, as Mr. Humphry has, they have already expressed their personal desire to put themselves to death when they feel that it is time for them to go.

It's selfishness. They don't want to suffer pain, they don't want to suffer anguish, they don't want to suffer at all, they just want to have everything they possibly can for the years in which they are "productive" and then they express the desire to kill themselves.

What do the churches feel about this?

I think the churches have to be, at this point, in a state of shock, and have not, to the best of my knowledge, done very much to speak out on the whole question of euthanasia.

In many states where pro-life movements have tried to fight off living-will legislation, we have seen an apathetic church. The true ramifications of this self-centered society have not dawned on the church. It comes down to the argument that if God gives life, only God can take life, and it is our responsibility to shepherd and protect our brothers and sisters while we are here on this earth. But preserving their lives simply is not of paramount importance in the churches.

Wouldn't we be better off if the churches had stayed out of the whole question completely?

I don't know that church leaders have any place in compromise. Church leaders who are involved in politics have mastered the art of politics, which is the art of compromise, and have forgotten that their primary responsibility is to the teachings of the church, the teachings of the Bible, and certainly not to please Democrats or Republicans or anyone but God.

If the churches remain uninvolved, they will be saying by silence that the mentality of death is not an issue, not their concern.

I believe that churches should be deeply involved but that their involvement should be without any compromise. Church leaders who uphold the teaching of God as stated in the Bible are good for America. But church leaders turned political pragmatists will destroy America.

Chapter 8

The Vocabulary of Death

Judie, the language used to defend abortion can be persuasive. For instance, being in favor of freedom to choose sounds like a good thing. What can you do about that?

For any particular cause to succeed, you must somehow frame the issue, change the language and attempt to have an impact on public opinion. The abortionists have been very successful in changing the language. A very popular word we see all over the place today is "choice"—there is even a credit card by that name.

Before the pro-death movement took over, we knew the word "choice" meant deciding which car we were going to buy, or what we would choose in the grocery store if there were several different brands.

But today the word "choice" is on a par with

the word "me." "Choice" often connotes selfishly deciding what's best for me—not selecting a bargain; not selecting what would be best for our family but rather selecting something by "choice" that is best for me as an individual. Me, the selfish person, "Choice," the exclamation of the selfish me. And, in accord with this eighties definition of "choice," the preborn baby certainly has no choice.

We have to answer the persuasive pro-death vocabulary with the facts. When NOW says a woman has a right to choose, what they don't say is that the woman has a right to choose to kill another human being. They never finish the sentence.

That gives quite a definition to the word "choice." How about the phrase "every child a wanted child"? That sounds reasonable.

To call a child—a human being—a commodity is exactly what that phrase does. It equates children with things. You might want a new car, you might want a loaf of bread different from the one you bought. But you certainly can't place a human being on the same level with a possession.

But that is what has happened. Our children have become property, things we can want or not want, and therefore it becomes easy for us as a society to look on preborn children and decide for ourselves what this child will or will not be able to achieve, and whether or not we even want the child. Thus, decisions are made to abort human beings.

Well, why should unwanted children be brought into the world?

We have to define what the word "wanted" means. It is an extremely emotional term. First, look at what happens in every pregnancy—between the sixth and eighth weeks, the mother will experience depression. I don't think that in any pregnancy the mother is happy every single moment for the entire nine months. There are times she wishes she wasn't pregnant. Does that make the child unwanted?

But supposing the pregnancy was a mistake and now the mother doesn't really want the baby. Won't she be more likely to abuse the baby?

No. Child abuse results from parents who expect too much from their children, or results from a heritage of child abuse—parents who were abused as children often turn around and abuse their own children. But child abuse is also more likely to occur with couples who desperately desire a first child and create a big set of expectations as to what this child will be like and how this child will behave. When the child can't live up to their expectations, they are more likely to be child abusers.

In fact, abortion doesn't prevent child abuse —it causes it! Not only is abortion itself child abuse in its worst form; abortion creates the mentality of death, of viewing children as a wanted or unwanted commodity. This mentality breeds child abuse.

But whether or not a mother "wants" her child, she has a responsibility to her baby. If she does not feel she can properly care for the baby, there are many families who desperately want children but cannot have them. Adoption offers the distressed pregnant woman the opportunity to provide her preborn baby a gift which killing that baby destroys.

Then we have to return to the foundation of the pro-life movement: faith. It is an argument that abortionists won't accept, but nevertheless, along with the founders of this country, we believe that life comes from God.

When Planned Parenthood talks about "unwanted" children they presume that they have a right to dispose of unwanted people any way they wish. They are not considering their accountability to God. On judgment day, they cannot excuse themselves of murder by saying a child was unwanted. How will they answer when God says, "*I* wanted that child"?

How about the statement "every woman has a right to control her own body"? That sounds reasonable, doesn't it?

I think that, within the law, all of us believe that we each have a right to control our own bodies —within certain limits. For example, I can't legally take drugs that will kill me. Within the law, I can't protect my body by willfully killing other people who happen to get in my way. There are a lot of things within the law that I cannot do even though I have, under the law, a certain degree of control over my body.

The same thing applies to a woman: It is true that she has a right to control her own body, but when she becomes pregnant, she has no right to control another individual's body, even though the individual resides in her womb.

Once she is pregnant, we are not talking about her body. We are talking about her body and the body of another human being who lives within her. The tragic result of this assertion that a woman has a right to control her own body is that the womb has become a war zone.

Another slogan I hear is that you don't have a right to impose your religious views on others. That again sounds somewhat reasonable. I don't want anyone imposing their religious views on me. What do you say about that?

Another human being, distinctly different from yourself, resides within your womb once fertilization occurs—that is not a religious belief. It is a biological fact.

No one in the pro-life movement is trying to impose a religious belief on anyone. Biology is on our side. Scientific knowledge is on our side. The very scientists who support abortion are the ones who also support *in vitro* fertilization, as we have already discussed, and they are the same ones who have told us that life begins at fertilization. That is a scientific fact, not a religious belief.

Along those same lines, I often hear that "you can't legislate morality." Isn't that true? You can't make things right or wrong just by passing a law.

Certain moral principles are not peculiar to any one religion. The right to life is one of these. The government must, among other things, defend the rights of its citizens. Laws to protect innocent human life do not *make* murder wrong—human beings have a *God-given* right to life, and laws *protect* that right.

Our founding fathers, for example, had much to say about this. George Washington stated in his farewell address to the nation: "Reason and experience both forbid us to expect that national morality can prevail in exclusion of religious principle." John Adams underscored this point by saying: "Our Constitution was made only for a religious and moral people. It is wholly inadequate for the government of any other."

How about "keeping legislators out of our bedrooms"? Even if the Constitution doesn't guarantee a right to privacy, we don't want Congressmen and Senators telling us what to do in our bedrooms, do we?

Abortions don't take place in bedrooms. And we're not looking for laws to regulate truly private matters. But abortion is not just a private matter— it always involves at least two people. Here again we have the idea that the right to privacy takes precedence over the right to life. When people talk about "keeping legislators out of our bedrooms," they're trying to imply that abortion is a natural, private part of sex. But killing is not a natural part of sex, and if they were to murder someone in the privacy of their own bedroom, they would be prosecuted under the law.

What about "quality of life"? The quality of life is important.

Sure it's important, but suppose we're talking about the quality of *your* life, and maybe I'm going to decide for you that your life isn't worth living. If you are in a car accident, for example, and wind up with the loss of both of your legs, it is possible in our society today that someone would say your quality of life is not good enough for you to be treated to the maximum extent possible, because your contribution to society probably will be less than it was before your accident. And according to the quality-of-life ethic, it might be decided that you should not be treated for other conditions that you suffer from because in the end you will not make an important contribution to society.

The danger, always, in a term like "quality of life" is who is going to determine what that means, and who will apply it to me? Is it possible that I will lose my life because someone else determines that my quality of life is not good enough?

Now suppose we go a step beyond that and say that, because of something that *might* happen to me some time in the future, someone else decides that my life won't be worth living if that event happens, and therefore is going to kill me now. Well, that is exactly what is happening to thousands of helpless babies. People are saying that their life would be so terrible that they'd be better off dead, so they go ahead and kill them even though they're not suffering at all!

Suppose your friend smokes cigarettes, and you think someday that friend may get cancer. You think of all the pain and suffering—what a horrible death! So you pull out a gun and shoot your friend.

Or the baby in your womb might grow up in poverty, or have a chance of developing some kind of disease, so you take a knife and cut the baby to pieces. That's abortion, justified by the quality-of-life ethic.

What about the terms "sexual freedom" or "reproductive freedom"?

This again reflects the idea that abortion is a natural, private part of sex. The people who are demanding "sexual freedom" or "reproductive freedom" aren't really asking for freedom to have sex or for freedom to reproduce. They're demanding the "right" to have sex, reproduce and then kill their offspring.

*How about "death with dignity"? That
sounds reasonable. Everyone wants to die with
dignity.*

Well, I suppose that everyone wants to die
with dignity, but the term itself, "death with dignity," is used by the proponents of active euthanasia
to describe the act of killing terribly ill or elderly
people. "Death with dignity" describes the kind of
death that they would administer by their own
hands. What we have is a movement to promote active killing, but in a camouflaged way. "Becoming
a victim" is called "dying with dignity."

*"Living wills" sound reasonable, and they are
very popular. What about "living wills"?*

"Living wills" are not popular among the
common people. They are popular among those
who advocate the killing of the elderly and the
terminally ill.

A living will is a death warrant. No one needs
to sign a piece of paper in order to die. From the
moment fertilization occurs, you and I and
everyone else are terminal. We are going to die.
Over 4,000 of us die every day before we ever leave
the womb, but the rest of us who are able to escape
the abortionists will die because the natural end of

life is death itself. So you certainly don't need to sign a document to assure yourself of the ability to die. The living will makes it possible for someone else to take your life before natural death occurs. The philosophy behind the living will assumes that someone else knows best; you "will" your life out of existence.

Another supposed virtue of abortion is that it will eliminate "defective" children. What do you have to say about that?

Well, I don't think I have ever met a perfect person. Every single one of us is handicapped in some way—some of us more severely than others, some of us more obviously than others, but none of us are perfect.

Again, we go back to "quality of life." Why is that term used? If that term is applied to newborn infants with certain treatable conditions, then many newborn infants' lives will be snuffed out simply because they are not perfect. But then who is perfect? None of us is perfect. Sure, there are people born with serious handicaps, even horribly deformed, but they still have a right to live.

I also hear that a fetus is not a person; an embryo is not a person; a zygote is not a person.

All of those terms are medical and biological words describing the baby during the very early stages of pregnancy. *Fetus,* for example, means "little one." *Zygote* is a medical and biological term applied to the brand-new human being, and *embryo* is yet another medical and biological term describing the baby.

Those terms, which belong to science, have been used to desensitize the American public. Once the American public accepts the dehumanization of the tiny person who exists in the womb, it is easier to argue in favor of the killing. These terms remove the humanity of the preborn child and place the preborn child on a plate as a thing that can be eliminated at will.

I hate being called, in reference to my own past, a zygote or a fetus. But if abortionists began to use the word "baby," more people would wake up to what abortion is all about. Being unfamiliar with medical and biological terms, many people interpret the labels *fetus, embryo* and *zygote* to mean that a child in the womb, especially one in the first months of pregnancy, is nothing but a blob of tissue.

What about "the product of conception"? What does that mean?

If a woman goes to an abortion clinic, she won't be told that they want to get rid of the baby growing inside of her. She'll be told that they will take out "the product of conception." Now anyone who has a grade-school education knows what conception produces: a baby. But by cloaking reality in an innocuous-sounding term, she, and maybe the abortionists, try to shield their consciences from the awful reality of what they're doing.

A pregnant woman isn't just going to have a baby; in truth, she already has one. But at an abortion clinic or referral center she will be told that if she doesn't want to have a baby, an abortion will take care of that, that she won't have one. Quite literally, that is true. But they're not taking away a baby she might have had at some time in the future—they're taking away the baby she already has growing inside her.

So a preborn baby is a person, but to justify the killing, we're being told, "No, there's no person there."

Yes. One hundred and thirty years ago, something similar was going on. Slaves were being defined as property, not as human beings, and this kind of thinking was upheld by the Supreme Court in the Dred Scott decision of 1857. Even though

Dred Scott, a runaway slave, had escaped to a state in which slavery was illegal, the court ruled that he was still property. As the now infamous Final Dred Scott Appeal stated (March 16, 1857): "The right of property in a slave is distinctly and expressly affirmed in the Constitution. The right of traffic in it, like an ordinary article of merchandise and property, was guaranteed to the citizens of the United States . . . and the government is pledged to protect it in all future time."

In our society today, the denial of personhood to preborn children who reside in the womb has resulted in mass killings. *Roe v. Wade* went further in its effects, however, than the Dred Scott decision because after the Dred Scott decision many of the victims were able to stand and fight and help secure their right to be recognized as human beings. They were not totally helpless.

However, preborn children are slaughtered by the millions and they are not able to form an army, they are not able to argue their case because they have no voice. They are dead.

What is the "squeal rule"?

In 1981, the Reagan administration proposed regulations to require that parents be notified after teenagers receive birth control pills or devices in school or in local birth control clinics. The individuals and organizations that provide birth control to children argued against the Reagan administration by saying that the government wanted birth control providers to "squeal" on teenagers. Use of this term makes it sound as if withholding information is good and releasing it is bad. It also presupposes that the government and Planned Parenthood have the teenagers' best interests at heart, and that parents do not.

If the vocabulary of death must be answered with facts, could you sum up the pro-life responses? What should we say when we hear the word "choice"?

We should respond with, "Choice—to kill a child."

What about the word "fetus"?

Fetus means "little one," appropriate for little children, especially little children in the womb.

"Product of conception"?

Product of conception equals the dead body of a brand-new human being.

"Right to privacy"?

The right to privacy means a woman's right to terminate the life of her new baby because it is inconvenient for her to have the baby.

"Sexual freedom"?

Sexual freedom is when man, unable to recognize the tremendous gift of human sexuality, cheapens sex so that it is nothing more than a commodity to be bought and sold.

"Quality of life"?

Quality of life is an excuse for one group in our society to effectively eliminate another.

"Every child a wanted child"?

That means kill the children we are too selfish to care for.

"A woman's right to control her own body"?

It really means a license for no self-control. By not controlling her sexual urges, she decides to destroy the body of her own child.

"Imposing your morality on me"?

Means saving someone else's life.

"You can't legislate morality."

Morality is note being legislated today because selfish interests deny moral absolutes.

"Let's keep the legislators out of our bedrooms."

The proper role of government is to defend and protect the people of this nation, including children who reside in the womb.

"Death with dignity"?

Means murder without penalty.

A "living will"?

A death warrant enabling a third party to prematurely end your life.

"Safe, legal abortion"?

Licensed, lethal child abuse.

Chapter 9

The Church and Abortion

All faiths must have respect for human life, right, Judie? Yet almost all churches and the Jewish and Islamic faiths seem silent or visibly weak in defense of life. What is the problem with the churches? Why aren't they involved?

I think one of the problems is that religious people in leadership positions have somehow forgotten that their main purpose as leaders of their flocks, so to speak, is to set absolute moral guidelines for people to follow. It is up to the leadership of the churches to declare what is right and wrong, without ever discussing any other possibility.

But today in the churches we hear so much about the gray areas with regard to so many of these issues that affect all of us as human beings. The leaders are afraid to condemn sin. The churches have grown weak because they are afraid to confront evil; they would rather dialogue than continue to preach what is right and wrong.

Why are the churches afraid to confront evil?

Many church leaders are desirous of protecting such trivial things as tuition tax credits and are fearful of IRS audits; because they are afraid of losing their tax-exempt status, they sometimes sit back and say nothing.

It's tragic in two ways. First, because their silence can be bought. The devil has found out their price for keeping quiet about abortion and other evils. Second, it's tragic because there is plenty the churches can do without jeopardizing their tax exemption.

I think too that a lot of church leaders have swallowed the twisted interpretation of separation of church and state that's making the rounds these days.

The United States was founded by people who were looking for religious freedom. It's true that not all persecution was left behind when they came to America, but there was a consensus among the founders that freedom of religion ought to be protected, to the point where they forbade the government to establish a state religion. The whole intent of this was to ensure that everyone could freely practice various faiths; tax exemption for churches was part of this—the government was prohibited from taxing churches because it could, if it chose, literally tax them to death. The whole idea was to prevent government interference in religion.

Nowadays, however, many people are talking as though the government should be hostile to any religion, rather than protecting them all equally, and they are saying that allowing the churches a voice on moral matters and not just doctrine is involving the churches in the government. They choose to overlook the fact that preaching morality is an integral part of both Jewish and Christian faiths. The job of religion in American always has been not just to teach doctrine—for the Jews to preach the coming Messiah or Christians to preach the divinity of Christ—but to preach morality, what is right and wrong.

Further, contrary to pro-abortion rhetoric, the American government has always had as its role the enforcement of morality. For almost two hundred years we had agreement among the American people that certain things—killing, stealing, lying under oath—were morally wrong and should be prohibited by law.

What it boils down to is that certain people no longer believe that killing is wrong, and they are using a distorted version of separation of church and state to eliminate the laws against killing, at least certain classes of people: the preborn, the elderly, the sick, the handicapped.

And in so doing they are trying to eliminate any religious influence in government?

Wrong. In 1961 the Supreme Court ruled (in *Torcaso v. Watkins*) that secular humanism is a religion, and the fact is that the religion of secular humanism has become, in practice, the unofficial religion of the United States.[18]

What is secular humanism?

In a nutshell, it's belief that humanity is the supreme being. Secular humanism declares that there is no God, that there is no creation of any kind, that mankind is continually evolving into a higher, refined, more perfected race, that nothing is objectively right or wrong, that we decide for ourselves what is right and wrong. In fact, secular humanists have a "creed" known as the Humanist Manifesto. Just as many formal religions have outlined their basic tenets of church teaching in a form easily understood, so too the secular humanists have their basic tenets.

Now, you won't find many people saying, "I'm a secular humanist," the way I say, "I'm a Catholic." For the most part, they don't have a church they go to, but, if you think about it, you will probably realize that you know quite a few people who believe the things taught by secular humanism. That is their faith.

How has it become the unofficial religion of the United States?

We've been talking about legalized killing. Do you think that legislators would vote for abortion funding, or court justices vote for abortion rights, if they believed in God, a God who forbids killing, who told us in the Bible that unrepentant murderers will end up in hell? It's plain that they are not afraid of God. The Bible says that fear of the Lord is the beginning of wisdom, and it's easy to see that many of our elected and unelected officials don't have even the beginning of wisdom. Why? Because of their practice of secular humanism!

The religion of secular humanism is also evident in the laws and policies having to do with education. Instead of religion being protected, prayer is forbidden on school property. Schools teach that humanity is a biological accident, that we have no idea how we got here, and for the most part educators are forbidden to teach anything else.

So we have our own government doing a good job of stamping out faith in God, maybe as good a job as the communist governments do, maybe better. Which brings us back to the churches.

Too many church leaders have accepted a government-encouraged role—teaching doctrine but not preaching morality. Not all of them, of course. But many of them are not telling people what's right and wrong, or if they are, they are not preaching reward and punishment. Instead of preaching hell for murder, some are telling their people, by their own example, that the worst thing you have to fear is losing your money, as in losing tax exemption, for example.

You're painting a picture of religious leaders abdicating responsibility.

We have no conviction coming forth from the churches. When they do preach morality, it is restricted by what the ministers, priests and rabbis perceive as their ability to get political. You will hear many church leaders talk about the killing of preborn innocent human beings as nothing more than a political issue.

And you're saying that abortion, which is

*called a social issue quite often today, really isn't a
social issue, is it?*

Of course it isn't. When you argue in the halls
of Congress about a tuition tax credit, nobody is
dying while your discussion goes on. Yet every day
when the discussion of abortion as a "social issue"
continues, 4,000 human beings are being annihilated in this country. It is certainly not a social issue.
It is a life-and-death question that must be
answered and it must be answered first in the
pulpit.

*While the pro-life movement seems to have
been led initially by Catholics, it has been joined in
the late seventies and early eighties by many different Protestant churches. What do you see in that?*

I think I see the pro-life movement becoming
truly pro-life. I see the Protestant churches joining
with the Catholic church, joining with the Jewish
groups, all together, not because they agree
doctrinally but because they see the reality of what
abortion is. They recognize that abortion is Satanic,
that abortion is only part of the overall problem
facing our society today, and that we must unite to
stop the devil from overcoming our entire nation.

And at some point in the future, after we have

returned our nation to God, we will then be able to go back to arguing among ourselves. But the unity coming forth by this recognition of evil as it exists in our society today is nothing but good for the pro-life movement.

It would be good for the church in general to have people of many faiths now working together, learning a little about each other's religion, who years ago probably wouldn't even have talked to each other.

Oh, that is right. I think there is a tremendous healing going on, but again it is going on among lay people. It is not because the leaders of the church have decided to return to teaching right and wrong with no buts about it. It is because the lay people have decided among the churches to get together and do everything possible to stop these heinous crimes from continuing in our country. The lay people still have little leadership from the churches, per se.

But isn't it true of any revolution, that generally change is brought about by the lay people, and not necessarily by the leadership?

I think that is one of the reasons the Civil War

was fought. People understood what was at stake. And that is what is going on today. People have had enough. And they are not waiting for some church leaders to rise up and tell them they are right. They know they are right and they are moving forward.

Do you think this unity will continue to grow within the churches? Do you think the day will come when they all will speak out with one voice and end the carnage?

I think ultimately it will take a spiritual revolution in America. We see now, for the first time, the same churches fighting pornography, fighting permissive sex education in the schools, fighting abortion, fighting all the causes of abortion, defending the right of children to pray in school. Together this enormous mass of people will ultimately change the law in our country, because they will ultimately themselves create a situation whereby people with religious convictions will be seated in our government and on the Supreme Court, and our country will once again be what I am sure George Washington and John Adams hoped it would be when they founded it many years ago.

Do you think that what is really needed is for the righteous to regain control of the churches?

No, I think that what is needed first, and what still hasn't happened, is that our country has to get down on its knees and seek God's forgiveness. The sin of abortion is not a sin just of our opposition; it is a sin of our nation. It is a sin for which all of us as human beings are accountable before God. And until this nation gets down on its knees, seeking God's will and asking for His forgiveness, nothing else that we do can possibly make a difference. We shouldn't stop working for the change, but we must be aware of our position before God.

Well, what can the church do about "Joe Sixpack," sitting down drinking beer, watching TV, mowing his lawn, playing golf—"the man on the street" who really doesn't care whether the sun rises tomorrow morning or not?

First, the churches have to preach repentance and judgment. We as a nation and as a church are guilty and even among those who haven't actively participated in or advocated abortion, few of us have done everythng in our power to stop it. Think of the story of the good Samaritan in the Bible; the robbers who beat the man and left him for dead were certainly wicked, but the men who passed him by on the road were guilty too.

We have to acknowledge that—abortion is a

sin and we're guilty. I think those who *have* done everything in their power to stop it are more convinced of that than anyone.

Second, the churches have to preach not just repentance but Christian solutions. It's simply not enough to say how bad abortion is, that it's a great shame. People have to hear about their own responsibility and what they can do.

I believe that abortion will be stopped when the people in every neighborhood in America believe that abortion is simply an unacceptable solution to any problem. And they must be willing to make personal sacrifices to help others less fortunate than themselves.

So, belief in God, belief in the sanctity and dignity of human life, but probably more important the practice that goes with that belief—is this what we need?

Oh, yes, and that is why our opposition makes so much headway in arguing against us. We have not yet as a movement made the real sacrifice to be there where a person is in trouble, not only during pregnancy, but at any point of development. Why are there so many minority children available for adoption and no white children? Because we, as a movement, have not delivered 100 percent. And until we do, we can't win.

Jesus said one of the greatest commandments is to love thy neighbor as thyself.

For the love of God.

If that were practiced, would this be over?

Oh, absolutely, there would be no discussion about abortion in our country if we practiced the second great commandment. We just don't. We choose to be more human than Godly because of the basic human temptation of putting self before others. Even those of us within the pro-life movement say that we are against abortion but at times we are unwilling to make the personal sacrifices needed to stop the carnage.

Chapter 10

Hard Cases

Judie, what about abortions necessary to save the life of the mother?

According to some studies done by obstetricians and gynecological organizations in this country in the last twenty years, we have had no case reported of an abortion performed to save the life of the mother.[19] However, by the word "abortion" we mean the intentional killing of the preborn child.

There are two non-abortion surgeries that always take the life of the preborn child. They are for conditions that would ultimately take the life of the mother as well. The first are pregnancies that occur in the fallopian tube—tubal pregnancies. A tubal pregnancy cannot continue because the baby cannot grow properly in the tube itself and the tubal pregnancy, if not ended, will ultimately kill the baby and the mother as well.

The second case is cancer of the uterus. If the cancer begins to spread, which it usually does, and the woman happens to be pregnant during this cancerous uterine condition, not only will the baby be killed by the cancer, but the mother will be too unless the cancer is removed. At the time of surgery, when the physician does what he can to remove the cancer, he will, of course, do everything he can to save the life of the preborn child if the pregnancy is far enough along. But if, in fact, the death of the baby is caused by the removal of the cancerous uterus, that is certainly not to be considered an abortion.

There are no other conditions still existing to-day that will cause the death of the mother if the pregnancy is carried to term. And in each of these cases, I repeat, the baby would be killed by the natural course of events if surgery were not performed.

How about pregnancies resulting from rape? Wouldn't carrying a rapist's child to term cause more psychological damage to the rape victim? After all, the rape victim didn't choose to have sex, let alone get pregnant, so isn't it only fair to let her have an abortion?

The actual incidence of pregnancy as the result of rape is 1 in 100,000 cases of rape. However, "rape," as has been the case with a lot of other words in our language, has come to be abused by the radical feminist movement. What we find, for example, in our research of the rape crisis centers that have been founded and funded by women's organizations is that they are simply another front group for abortion referral and abortion promotion and, in fact, in many cases the performance of abortion itself.[20]

It is just another hinge upon which the radical feminist movement has been able to hang its hat, collect taxpayer money and continue to encourage the destruction of marriage. Many times we are told in the media, for example, that a woman was "raped" because she had an argument with her husband either directly after or directly before sexual intercourse within the marriage.

And we know that is probably not the case. But in their continued efforts to destroy marriage, the radical feminist movement has made an effort to portray husbands as raping their wives. This argument makes it easier for wives to leave their husbands, get a divorce and in many cases obtain an abortion.

Planned Parenthood distributes a booklet called *Let's Tell the Truth About Abortion*, and on page 14 they describe rape in a brand-new way:

"Let us say a married woman is forbidden by her church to use contraception but the family can't feed another child so she refuses sex but is forced by her husband. Is this rape? How about the divorced husband who comes to visit and forces his ex-wife just to prove he can. Is this rape? How about the case in which a 20-year-old man has intercourse with a drunken 15-year-old too silly not to drink and too drunk to fight him off. Is this rape?"

All of these scenarios presented by Planned Parenthood, through their Fight Back Press, are designed to encourage removal of the present legal definition of rape and to make it easier for a woman to claim that she has been raped, no matter what the circumstances might actually be. In all of the cases described above, a criminal forcible rape did not occur nor could the woman in any of these cases bring charges of criminal rape against her boyfriend or her husband.

In the case of criminal rape we have to understand first that the traumatization of the woman's body is so severe that pregnancy rarely occurs as the direct result of a rape, or as the direct result of a forcible incestuous relationship.

However, if a child does exist in the womb, the child is a non-aggressor. The child has not perpetrated a crime and should not be made to suffer.

From what we know about the psychological implications of abortion, it would seem to me that we are only compounding the psychological complications of rape, or a forcible act of incest, by adding to them the forcible destruction of an innocent human being in the womb of a woman who is already a victim. If we did this, we would have a case on our hands of multiple psychological side effects, which would in the end do more damage to the woman who had the abortion than they would if she had chosen to carry the child to term.

What do you do in the case of incest?

Most cases of incest are between stepfathers and stepchildren, and major causes of this are our promiscuous society and the high rate of divorce and remarriage.

There are no statistics on pregnancy resulting from incest because it is always within a family and rarely reported. Now that incest has become a frequent subject of television movies and radio and television talk shows, I think there will be a terrible increase in incest in this country.

Of course, the media will not take the blame, but will simply say that things have always been this bad and that thanks to them it is finally being discussed openly.

But as to pregnancy from incest, it is certainly rare if the incest involved physical trauma. Even if it did not, the baby is just another victim of the situation, and certainly the least deserving of punishment, especially capital punishment!

With sperm banks and their anonymous donors, I don't think we have yet begun to see incest as bad as it's going to get. All of the problems of intermarriage may surface when blood relatives unwittingly marry each other. This kind of thing has already happened, but I definitely believe it's going to get worse.

What about children born with severe handicaps? Shouldn't some just be allowed to die?

If we took each case on its own merits, which used to be the common practice, we would find that doctors are well equipped to help parents determine the proper treatment for handicapped children. The medical knowledge available today, which is much more than even ten years ago, is enough for doctors to make sound decisions if they are guided by moral principles.

The problem is not with babies who are born with a terminal illness. Some infants are not going to survive no matter what is done. And those conditions are readily recognized by a medical staff trained in neonatal care.

The problem is that some members of the medical and legal professions are arguing that even some infants with treatable conditions should receive no medical treatment, or even no food and water! They base their argument on their "quality of life" standards, by which they endow themselves with the right to determine that at some time a child's life will not be worth living and that therefore they have the right to withhold treatment, and/or food and water from a baby.

One of the best-known cases in recent years was the baby born in Indiana who had Down's Syndrome and a condition that required tracheal surgery for the baby to be able to eat. Neither of these conditions was terminal. However, the parents and physicians agreed not to treat the infant and to let the baby starve to death. That took six days. Meanwhile, other parents of children with Down's Syndrome, parents who knew the problems of raising children with the disease, were offering to adopt the baby.

But a judge refused to prevent the doctors and parents from starving their baby, not even long enough for others to adopt him.

Another case involved "Baby Jane Doe." She was born with spina bifida, and again the parents and doctors decided not to treat the baby. Spina bifida is not a terminal illness, so here too we have doctors and the baby's own parents determining that a life is not worth living. However, even babies want to live—they have just as strong an instinct for self-preservation as you or I—and Baby Jane Doe was doing so well without treatment that the doctors and parents relented and performed the necessary surgery to correct the spinal deformation.

These two cases inspired regulations by the federal government to insure that newborn infants are not denied treatment where there is any hope, and especially to insure that all babies are fed. But these regulations have met with opposition from doctors and the courts, and there is still no effective legal safeguard for the lives of the handicapped.

How about the elderly? Some people hang on, suffering, for months or even years. Isn't it merciful to let them die?

As with handicapped infants, some conditions are not treatable, and anything the doctors can do is useless. But the danger is that a lot of people consider themselves qualified to decide when someone else's life is no longer worth living. We must not accept killing as a solution to suffering, much less for poverty or inconvenience. Society has already approved of murder in the womb; society is looking very strongly at approving of murder in the nursery; and now society is discussing the acceptability of killing a loved one, not because the loved one necessarily wants to be put out of misery but because it is easier on the conscience of the one who is observing the pain and suffering if he no longer has to observe it.

Those are simply not decisions that the legal system or this society should be making, because they are all decisions that place society above God, and completely devalue the human being's intrinsic worth to society.

Pro-life people are all for saving babies, but what are you doing for the children who are already here?

There is a tremendous range of services available, such as shepherding homes, that are growing in number every day. These are homes where a young woman can live, not just while she is pregnant, but until she gets back on her feet, until she can get her life in order, until she can acquire the education necessary to carry on a productive job in the marketplace and take care of her child by herself.

I think one problem has been not just within the pro-life movement but within society as a whole. Where the pro-life movement has asked repeatedly for assistance from the community, the anti-life movement has been there offering the solution of death rather than the sacrifice necessary for a family to defend life and protect that life, both before and after birth.

What do you do for the parents who have a handicapped child with severe birth defects who go ahead and have the baby but don't want to raise it? Do pro-lifers do anything for children like that?

Yes, in fact, in each case where we are made aware of the birth of a severely handicapped newborn infant, there is always a multitude of families ready and waiting to adopt these children, if the parents find that they would rather give the child up for adoption than try to care for the child and come up with the money for the medical expenses, which in some cases can be astronomical.

In the case of the family who decides to keep the child and do everything humanly possible for the child, then I think financial assistance and programs of rehabilitation and treatment for the baby are necessary. It often involves more help than an individual or a few individuals can give. This help may come from the government or the church or both, thus making it possible for the parents of such a baby not to have to worry about money, but to devote themselves to the care of the child.

What is your answer for the epidemic of teenage pregnancy? You may save the babies, but once teenagers start having sex they're not going to stop.

That's wrong. Planned Parenthood, Ann Landers and Abigail Van Buren are always saying that, but it's not true. If you read between the lines, they're saying that sex outside of marriage, even though it's wrong, is so great that once anyone has tasted the forbidden fruit they're not going to stop. The fact is that very few women find sex outside of marriage fulfilling in any way. In most of those kinds of relationships, the man is just using the woman, or in terms of teenagers, the boy is using the girl. Although claiming to liberate women, the people who promote adultery and fornication are really denying to women the stability of marriage. They are making it easy for men and women to get physical pleasure from sex without accepting any responsibility. This is not what most women want, and it's not what anybody needs.

There is an answer, and that is chastity. But it has to be taught. Planned Parenthood, Ann Landers and Abigail Van Buren tell parents not to bother trying to teach teenagers a better way, and they tell teenagers not to listen. However, any teenage girl who has been having sex outside of marriage, especially if she's had a baby but no husband, or worse, had an abortion, knows that sexual sin isn't all it's cracked up to be. And maybe her boyfriend (if she's pregnant, probably her ex-boyfriend) has started to realize that too. They'll both be ready to listen to a better way, God's way. But their parents have to teach them. And of course it's better yet to be teaching them chastity before they become promiscuous. That is the solution to promiscuity among teenagers.

Remember, the epidemic is adolescent promiscuity, not adolescent pregnancy.

What about artificial birth control?

As we discussed earlier, most forms of artificial birth control are harmful, none are 100% effective, and many of them terminate the life of the baby.

But, particularly in the area of teenage sex, they are not helping. Promiscuity among teens has simply skyrocketed, along with the incidence of venereal disease. And, as I pointed out before, the "sexual freedom" supposedly achieved by the use of birth control is just an illusion.

A careful examination of the AIDS epidemic confirms the fact that today promiscuous sex, even with the use of artificial birth control, leads to lethal disease. AIDS is terminal.

Furthermore, as use of birth control has become widespread the divorce rate has gone up too. I think this is partly due to the harm done by birth control to the sexual relationship in marriage. It encourages husband and wife to look at each other more as objects to satisfy their own desires; it separates the natural aspects of fatherhood and motherhood from sex.

What about an eleven-year-old who becomes pregnant? Wouldn't it be safer for her to have an abortion?

An eleven-year-old has a very good chance of delivering a normal, healthy child. She may deliver a smaller child because her womb is smaller, but she can deliver normally.

Because her womb is so immature, however, if it is invaded by the steel instruments and drugs during an abortion, not only will the baby die, but many times the young lady will be damaged for life.

What would you do when prenatal testing shows a likelihood of severe birth defects?

In the first place, we have no right to kill anyone just because they are impaired in some way. If you grant someone the right to determine that a baby's life should end because the baby is impaired, how do you know that person won't turn around and decide *you* are impaired? That may sound like an exaggeration, but you can see it happening already with the elderly and with newborn infants.

Second, the tests, such as amniocentesis and chorionic villus biopsy, are dangerous in themselves and are not 100% accurate. They too often result in abortion of perfectly healthy babies who, according to the tests, might have been impaired. In other cases, they harm a baby who was perfectly all right before the test. When tests don't offer an opportunity for treatment within the womb, all they do is encourage more killing.

What is the pro-life answer for not being against nuclear war or for not being directly involved in the peace movement?

The devastation that has already occurred by the killing of over twenty million children in our country is so serious that there isn't anyone in the anti-war movement who should ever accuse the pro-life movement of being anything but totally pro-life. We have tried to prevent the killing of innocent human beings who live in the war zone commonly known as the womb. That is where the need is most immediate. Of course, many pro-life people, perhaps most, are active in other areas besides pro-life. But to answer the crying need, we have organizations devoted specifically to protecting the preborn, helping mothers, providing for babies' needs and so forth. And that is no different from what other concerned people do. There are organizations whose main interests are anti-war, etc. You might say to them, "You may prevent deaths in a war, but how are you going to feed the people whose lives you save?"

To state it another way, how can one oppose nuclear weapons if one is not born? How can one assist the homeless if one is not born? The war known as abortion must be stopped!

Pro-lifers want a baby to live in the womb, but they don't specifically oppose capital punishment. Why not?

The preborn child is in every case innocent. He did not ask to reside in the womb, no matter what the cause of the pregnancy, even such a violent cause of pregnancy as a rape. The baby is always an innocent victim. If a man breaks a law and is sentenced to death, it is because he has violated someone else's rights; in many cases he has destroyed a human being.

The pro-life movement is in the business of defending all innocent human beings, not criminals who have broken the laws of this country. The criminal sentenced to death can in no way be equated with the preborn child who innocently tries to reside in his mother's womb.

How about poor people? You don't want them to have abortions, but what do you do to help them?

As I pointed out already, the endangered right to life requires such effort that we have organizations devoted to protecting and recovering that right. But among the ranks of the pro-life movement there are literally thousands of people who volunteer in soup kitchens, who deliver meals on wheels, who spend hours every day caring for handicapped children and intervening with families where there are difficulties because of a handicap or because of a terminally ill person. Because of those human actions, people are drawn into the war against abortion.

Each action to protect or assist the poor and the downtrodden is an action that will rarely be recognized by the media or the government, or by anyone else, because these people silently give of themselves in very unselfish ways.

Shouldn't pro-life people be for gun control?

The pro-life movement is composed of conservatives, of liberals, of a lot of people who have various views on the subject of gun control. I don't frankly believe that gun control has much to do with the arbitrary killing of 4,000 innocent children every day in America.

Pro-life people are protecting and nurturing lives of others, starting in their own families with their own children and then reaching out into the community to do everything they can to make life easier and more loving, just as Christ would have them do.

Chapter 11

Tying It All Together

You have said a number of times that abortion is more than just one thing. How do you tie in the various related concerns? For instance, pornography, homosexuality, AIDS, sex instruction in the classroom, birth control clinics in schools themselves—you've expressed concern about these. What ties them all together?

The common thread that runs among pornography, homosexuality, sex instruction, birth control clinics in the schools, abortion on demand and euthanasia is a complete disrespect for the human being as a distinctly unique and unrepeatable miracle. These assaults on human persons treat individuals simply as things on the same level as car racing, gambling or drinking. They are all related to a decline in moral values in America.

*I know they have sex instruction in schools
from kindergarten right on up through high school.
What effect does that have on abortion,
euthanasia, the death mentality?*

Sex instruction is an outgrowth of secular
humanism. One must differentiate basic sex education and sex instruction. Basic sex education is
education in biology, the dangers of venereal
disease and the functions of the human body—a
course that would perhaps take one half of one
semester during one school year.

What we have today, rather than the basic sex
education information, is an entire course that
takes twelve years and deals with the devaluation of
human sexuality and a cooperative devaluation of
the human being as a unique individual. Sex instruction is part of a broader secular humanistic
program that teaches children such things, for example, as the acceptability of death, or the assump-
tion that we can eliminate the weaker members of
society, by such games as "lifeboat."

The connection between sex instruction, death
education and other such courses which deal with
the devaluation of human life is the teaching of a
religion—secular humanism." We are told that in
the public school system no religious values are
taught. In truth, humanist values are taught while

Judaeo-Christian values are not.

People and kids are going to go out and have sex anyway. What are you going to do about that?

First of all, let's examine sex instruction programs in the classroom. In 1965 the federal government began funding sex instruction programs in the classroom. A study by the Alan Guttmacher Institute, the research arm of the Planned Parenthood Federation of America, showed that over the first ten years of taxpayer-funded permissive sex instruction in the classroom, the abortion rate among teens increased by over 225%, and the suicide rate among teens and the venereal disease rates among teens both escalated at dramatic rates.

What this proves is that the anti-life movement in its efforts to dehumanize human sexuality has made it is easier for teenagers to accept the killing of a preborn child than it is for them to accept self-restraint and chastity. The answer to the problem is that we must start teaching proper values. We must teach that sex is a valuable gift from God, not a cheap experience.

Is the dramatic increase in AIDS, syphilis, gonorrhea, herpes and other venereal diseases due to permissive sex instruction?

We can't just blame sex instruction in the classroom. There is a long list of factors.

First, there is the Playboy Foundation and their repeated dehumanization of women.

Additionally, there is the outright use of children in pornographic materials that are sold in any of the so-called adult bookstores in this country. There are movies being shown under the rating of PG-13. Many of these films are really pornography on the screen. Then there are televised pornographic rock videos and, of course, afternoon and evening soaps.

These things, combined with permissive sex instruction, have led society to a point where even such things as "alternative lifestyles," homosexuality and lesbianism, are portrayed to children in the same light and with the same value as family life where the mother and the father marry first and then have children.

In a situation like this it is the young people who suffer while many adults are propagating their own beliefs from a very selfish point of view, never caring at all about the future of youth.

I can name two other common threads running through the fabric of disrespect for human beings, human life and human sexuality. They are government funding and Planned Parenthood.

Federal and state governments unfortunately

provide lavish funding for both direct activities, such as abortion and abortion referrals, and for "education," that is, propaganda in favor of promiscuity, birth control, abortion, homosexuality and pornography. The "education" is often sponsored by Planned Parenthood with government support.

Planned Parenthood's permissive sex instruction programs have been accepted into many schools, even supposedly Christian ones. These courses comprise a twelve-year indoctrination. They do their best to replace traditional values instilled at home with a new set of values of their own devising. They openly suggest that neither parents nor churches have any business telling children not to have sex. They teach that "responsibility" means having sex with anyone you want to as long as no pregnancy results. They teach that if, by chance, a pregnancy results from this promiscuity, then there is always abortion.

Planned Parenthood teaches that oral sex, anal sex, homosexuality and anything else you may want to try is perfectly all right.

By the time students complete twelve years of sex instruction under the auspices of Planned Parenthood, they will have instilled in them a disrespect for human life, a casual attitude about sex, and a contempt for authority, religion and traditional values.

Another aspect of government funding for Planned Parenthood is that it is virtually worldwide. International Planned Parenthood works closely with the United Nations Fund for Population Activities, and, in countries with less freedom than we have, they have supported programs of forced sterilization and forced abortion.

They believe it is cheaper to sterilize women and men of the Third World than to invest in farm equipment and agricultural methods that will feed the people. All of the scare tactics that have been used in the past in the American press by the Hugh Moore Fund are found today in the discussion of such countries as Ethiopia.

Yet in Ethiopia they export food while people are starving to death simply because the people oppose a communistic form of government.

On an international scale, there has been an elitist movement setting the agenda. I don't want to call it a conspiracy because it's been going on in the open for close to a century.

But nevertheless there has been active promotion of death as a solution to the world's problems, and naturally it's packaged in a way that sounds humane and attractive. We talked about this in the chapter on the mentality of death. It involves cloaking the reality of killing, wrapping it up in nice terms. And it involves persuading people that it is necessary to give away their freedom, for example by chiseling away at the right to life. What makes it worse is that it's generally being done by very wealthy people, who instead of using their wealth to help people emerge from poverty are using it to promote their solution: death for the unwanted.

It's the work of the devil being displayed in a way we never expected to see in our lifetimes.

Part II

Questions and Answers
With
Paul Brown

Founder of
ALLPAC

Chapter 12

Politics and the Press

Why should a pro-life person be involved in politics?

Well, there are many solutions to the abortion problem. Perhaps one of the quickest fixes, on a temporary basis, is a political solution. In Congress, there are representatives elected to the House every two years and senators elected every six years. Some of these are very strong advocates and proponents of abortion. Pro-lifers, if they learn to work smart, and pick out a few of these people, can have an impact on their reelection. They can provide three to five percent of the vote and they can help change a close election and throw a bad guy out of office.

What if a person doesn't know anything at all about politics?

They can learn. Politics isn't really that difficult to understand. All you really have to learn is where a candidate, or an incumbent member of the House or Senate, or the President, stands on the issues of life and death.

How can I find that out?

It is very simple, and there are many ways to start. You can contact American Life League or ALLPAC. You can find out about your representative's voting record. You can write a letter to the politician who represents you—they are usually very honest on this particular issue. If your representative doesn't give you a straightforward answer, you can read between the lines to find out.

Just ask quite frankly, "Are you for or against abortion? How do you vote on the abortion issue? I want to know." The politician will generally respond and let you know exactly where he stands.

If I want to get involved in political action, what should I do?

All fifty states have pro-life organizations that are involved politically. Often it is possible with grassroots campaigning to swing an election and unseat an anti-life representative, governor or other elected official. But I also urge that you join a national pro-life political organization, because there is strength in numbers and it is possible to put that strength to work in a few crucial elections across the country. By concentrating on elections where we know we can make a difference we can change the makeup of the House of Representatives or the Senate.

Local organizations have a job to do, but they are sometimes too small and weak to have a great effect, and they may devote a lot of time and effort trying to remove from office someone who is strongly entrenched politically.

What about my own community? Will elections on my city council make a difference?

Every election is important, be it for dogcatcher, city council, mayor, county commissioner, state representative, governor, right on up the line. Each election is important.

But you can't win in all elections. You have to be a realist to some degree and realize that there are times when someone you don't like happens to be in office because he or she is too powerful to be defeated. Then you should put your efforts into other areas, such as education to build up your basic, grassroots strength. Once you build that I think you can beat anybody.

You called politics a temporary solution to the problem. What effect would politics have one way or the other on abortion?

Through political action we can affect federal funding of abortion, that is, taxpayer support of abortion. We can help curtail these funds to a certain degree. In the long run, politics will never solve the abortion problem. That is a matter of education and of people respecting the sanctity and dignity of human life.

What is all the talk about a Human Life Amendment?

The Paramount Human Life Amendment would protect all innocent human beings from the moment of fertilization onward without regard to age, health, or condition of dependency. This would ensure that nothing in the Constitution would be construed to mean that there is such a thing as a right to abortion. It would eliminate any basis for the Supreme Court, or any other court, to rule in favor of abortion rights.

But, for the time being, I think the Human Life Amendment is pie in the sky. I think there will be no Human Life Amendment in the near future. There will be no effective Human Life Amendment for a long time to come unless and until we educate the public on the issue of abortion itself—the actual killing, the murder of tiny little children.

Once people come to realize that abortion is wrong, then we can have laws to support our positions. But until we reeducate and change the minds and hearts of the American public and make them proponents of life, an amendment really wouldn't matter. If we had an amendment today there would probably be just as many abortions tomorrow as there were the day before, because society does not have a basic respect for human life.

Once I become aware of how local and state politicians stand on abortion, how can I possibly inform all my friends and neighbors if I don't have a large amount of money to spend on informing them?

Money is one thing the pro-life movement has never really had, as far as politics or anything else is concerned. So our strength is not money, our strength is motivating people. You contact your friends, your relatives and members of your church, and get them involved, get them started.

You have to remember that no great cause in

this country ever succeeded by being in the majority to start with. There was always a small minority that grew and built a solid grassroots base and eventually overcame because they educated the people around them.

So you can start in your neighborhood; you should start in your neighborhood. You should start with your neighbor, your best friend, converting them step by step. When your little part adds to all those other little parts that are being done all over the United States, eventually we will have an army for life.

Paul, we want to get organized. Can we do so with the aid of the media?

One or two people, which is really all it takes to start a local organization, can make inroads with the press as long as you remember always to be factual, brief and friendly.

Further, groups like ALLPAC and American Life League can provide you with material that will make the job of educating your community as well as your politicians easy and enjoyable.

Suppose the press, in my area, is totally anti-life. They never publish a letter to the editor when I write one. What can I do about that?

Well, there are a number of things you can do with the press. First, you have to understand the press. Most members of the press who are pro-abortion take that position because pro-life people have not educated them. They have never really heard the pro-life side. Take the person from the newspaper or television station to lunch. Befriend a member of the press. Don't attack them. Don't go after them personally. Try your best in your own way to educate them.

If you have friends who advertise in the newspaper, maybe that is one way of influencing the paper to at least present the pro-life story on an equal footing with the pro-abortion view. You would be surprised how just a few phone calls to a newspaper can change the management's opinion.

You told me not to make an enemy of the members of the press. If I get a lot of my friends to join me in criticizing the newspaper in my community, won't they turn us off and never pay any attention to us again?

Listen, I am not recommending that you bash heads. I am simply suggesting that advertisers can influence management by pointing out that a balanced view of any issue is far better than a one-sided report. It makes sense that those responsible for providing news would accept constructive criticism. Never stoop to personal attacks. That kind of behavior will not benefit the preborn child and it will, as you point out, alienate members of the media.

Further, it doesn't hurt for members of the press to know you are on different sides, where that is really the case. Even when they have totally opposing viewpoints to yours, you can accomplish a great deal by befriending them. Again, you have to understand where they are coming from. Most of them have their own opinions about us, based on their perception of us as fanatical crusaders, but they are also sometimes quite open to objective things. Most papers will print letters representing opposing points of view.

Make it a point to provide good, but brief, educational material to those you learn to know. By doing this, in addition to familiarizing them with your group's activities, you will build credibility and provide knowledge and understanding.

If I want to get my message out to the public through the press, how can I do that effectively?

Well, first, do not call a press conference and start preaching about the evils of abortion.

Why not?

Because they are not going to listen to you. They are not going to listen to anyone who preaches. The press is going to come to you when you offer them something they can print. One of the best ways to get press is to announce a picket of a local abortion clinic, or to announce that you are targeting a certain candidate and you are going to defeat him in the next election.

The press is news-oriented. They expect you to provide them with the who, what, when, where and why of the story you wish them to cover. When you provide this information, document your statements, and make the message brief, you will have done the media's work for them, and you will get coverage.

If I want to write a letter to the editor of my local newspaper, how long should it be? What should it say?

Letters to the editor should not exceed 150 to 200 words. In fact, I think 100 words is probably plenty. If your newspaper has a stated limit, observe that limit. Make each word count. You want to send a letter that is not too long or preachy, but one that expresses your opinion.

And writing letters to the editor is one of the best ways to get a free ad, so to speak, and express your own pro-life viewpoint. Furthermore, politicians pay attention to letters to the editor because they reflect public opinion. Maybe you can't afford to buy an ad in the newspaper, but by sending a letter dealing with certain topics it will get printed.

Each time a paper carries a story which does not present the pro-life view, you have an opportunity to express that view in a "letter to the editor." But you have to be awfully careful to know what you are talking about. Consult with your pro-life group about just what you should write. If you need to, contact American Life League; order one of our many publications.[21]

If I find out that a local or national politician is anti-life and I write a letter to the editor explaining what his position on abortion is, do I have a good chance of getting it printed?

You have a good chance if you are straightening the record out, if that politician has been putting up a shield and claiming that he is on both sides of the street and you can document that he is on the anti-life side. Then you have a good chance of getting it printed, especially if you say that you will work in the next election to defeat this official.

If I find out that my local politician is anti-life and I go to my minister and he tells me that he can't get involved in politics, what can I tell him?

One of the greatest reasons that we have abortion on demand today is ministers and priests and rabbis saying they can't get involved in politics. You have to get your minister involved in politics but first you have to educate him.

He has a right to express his opinion even in the pulpit. By law he cannot say the church stands this way or the church stands that way, for or against a particular politician. But he can say that he personally feels that because of the horrible voting record and the horrible anti-life stand of candidate A and because of the good stand of candidate B, that he personally is going to vote for candidate B. By making this kind of statement, the minister does not jeopardize the church's tax status. He is within his rights under the Constitution, and in fact, he has a moral obligation to make these facts known in the manner I have suggested.

My congressman writes and tells me that he is against abortion, but he continues to vote in favor of funding for organizations like Planned Parenthood. Is he pro-life?

Many politicians unfortunately are masters of the English language in that they can answer a question without ever answering a question and totally confuse you with the answer. The only guide you have to judge a politician is how he votes. His voting record is public information. It is available to anyone who requests it. Check his voting record, check him out.

Ask him questions in writing, and when he gives you a very bland answer or a no-answer letter, send back another letter demanding a specific answer. The chances are that your letter was answered by a clerk who doesn't even know or care where the politician stands. So be forceful and keep writing, persistently demand that the politician say exactly where he stands or, more importantly, how he votes.

Now, on the subject of Planned Parenthood funding, your congressman may have a different, but common, problem. Most politicians do not know just how big the abortion problem is. There are some pro-life congressmen who vote consistently against taxpayer funding of abortion, who co-sponsor human life amendments, who stand with us four-square, yet they may not have taken the time to understand Planned Parenthood and its love afffair with death.

It becomes a matter of education. They have

to learn that groups like Planned Parenthood are the chief proponents of abortion on demand in this country. Politicians will not accept this fact easily because they are accustomed to hearing the terms "birth control" and "population control" in the context of "caring solutions."

But until the public, until their own constituents actually educate them through repetition, they are not going to change. It is up to the pro-lifers living in the congressional district or in the Senate candidate's state to come forth and educate that politician. Once you have helped him, true pro-life politicians will change their ways. Many have in the past.

You said there are pro-life groups in every state. How can I be sure the group I join is really going to represent me?

Some "pro-life" groups refuse to count votes in favor of Planned Parenthood as part of politicians' voting records. Some are afraid to be against Planned Parenthood because they are ambivalent about the real causes of abortion as they have been discussed in this book (e.g., promiscuity, sex instruction, etc.). They don't like to rock the boat. The pro-life movement became successful because we stepped out in faith. You cannot stand in the middle. If you are a pro-lifer, you have to be 100% pro-life or you are not pro-life at all. There is no compromise on human life.

If a pro-life group doesn't take positions against population control, birth control for teenagers, abortion and euthanasia, then it isn't really pro-life.

You have to ask a few questions. Number one, "Do you truly believe in the sanctity and dignity of human life? Is life sacred?" Also, "Is God the real Commander-in-Chief of the pro-life movement?"

If they hesitate, be very suspicious. I think that some groups have their own agendas involved. It is very important for pro-life people to know exactly who they are supporting and why. If someone tells you that this is a civil rights movement and not a sanctity-of-life movement, be suspicious. They are not involved in this thing to bring a solution to the problem; they are involved simply to end surgical abortion—which will never solve this problem.

Politics, I am told, is the art of compromise, and you have just said that there can be no compromise on human life. How can abortion be a political issue?

It is a very difficult issue for the politician. In Congress, the main action is compromise. You are correct in saying, "Politics is the art of compromise." But politicians run into a strange creature when they run into a pro-lifer, because we have to tell them, "No compromise. No, we are not going to give you 10 babies to kill, or 50 babies, or 1,000, or 10,000, or 500,000." We have to be firm by saying that all life is sacred, all innocent life must be protected.

The day we compromise on our side, the day we give them a baby here or a baby there, we have lost the battle. So we can't compromise with the politicians; we must educate them. They deal in compromise on every other topic and that's fine. Water for South Dakota, a housing project for Brooklyn—these entail compromise, scratching one another's backs. But human life is sacred and can never be compromised. Pro-lifers can never give in.

If I become involved in pro-life political action, my friends are going to say that I have become a part of the New Right. Is that correct?

That is terribly incorrect. But it is a favorite slogan of the press and it is a statement that was made a number of years ago by the abortionists who set out to tie the pro-life movement to the so-called New Right.

Now, there are many areas we can work on in coalition with other groups. We can support the same legislation as long as it is protecting preborn children. We can work together as long as no compromise is involved.

In recent history there was the example of Democratic Senator John Durkin in New Hampshire, who was 100% with the pro-life movement. The New Right opposed his reelection while pro-lifers stood by him. Unfortunately, he lost.

The main question is, is the candidate pro-life? Whether he carries a liberal Democrat or a conservative Republican label is totally immaterial. If he is 100% pro-life, then you should back him.

Now, if we have two candidates who are pro-life, we should wish them both well and decide to work in either campaign. Our resources are few, and should be spent on races where there is a difference in position between candidates, and where we can make the difference for the babies.

If I become involved in politics, some of my friends will accuse me of forcing my religious views into the arena of political action where they don't belong. How do I answer that?

It is a matter of morality versus immorality. Either immorality is forced down our throats by elected officials supported by someone else, or we support candidates who vote for morality. Someone is going to win and someone is going to lose.

The world is made up of good and evil. We have to take our stand; we have to bring God back to the Constitution; we have to make the motto "In God We Trust" not just a little bit of writing on the dollar bill, but something real for America.

What problems should I watch out for in pro-life political action?

Well, Potomac Fever is one of my favorites (the Potomac River runs by the District of Columbia). Many people are well-meaning and well-intentioned in whatever they do and whatever they say back in their own communities, yet once they have been elected, once they move to Washington, D.C., they catch the "fever." The "fever" is being top dog on the street. The "fever" is being very important. For example, a politician picks up a newspaper and he reads his name. He immediately believes that he is very important and, sadly, at that point he is suffering from what could be a terminal case of "Potomac Fever."

I have always felt that pro-lifers should do all they can to get their own names and their organizations' names but especially the facts about the killing of babies into the paper. That is fine, and the more they can do it the better off we are because it is spreading our message.

But the day you get your name in the paper and you run out and buy the newspaper and start showing it to your friends, and tell them that it is your name in the paper that is important and not the issue, then you would do the pro-life movement a favor by taking a back seat.

Pro-life political action doesn't seem as strong as it used to be.

You have to put the pro-life movement into perspective. The pro-life movement became successful in the late seventies because pro-lifers said, "We are going to defeat candidates A, B and C." Regardless of what the press said—and no one really believed us—we *did* go out and beat candidates A, B and C. We were successful in spite of ourselves. We were successful because we believed we could accomplish the impossible. Today some pro-life political action leaders don't believe!

If we leave it up to God, does that mean we cannot compromise under any circumstances?

In life-and-death issues, there can be no

compromise. If we compromise we have sold our own souls. If we compromise, we have sold everything we are supposed to stand for. There can't be, never will be, a compromise when dealing with human life.

Don't even pro-life politicians sometimes think more of their political affiliation than about the lives of preborn babies?

That's one of the hard facts of life that pro-life groups must learn to accept. Many good pro-life politicians are first and foremost politicians. Pro-lifers have to recognize the fact that if a Republican who is anti-life is running for office against a pro-life Democrat, pro-life Republicans will work for that anti-life Republican.

It is a hard fact for us to accept, but we have to deal with the reality of the mattter. Some day, by working hard, we might change it.

(Please turn the page for important information about contacting the President and Congress.)

Addresses for writing to the president, your
senators and your congressman or
congresswoman:

The White House
Washington, DC 20500
Phone (202) 456-1414

U.S. Senate
Washington, DC 20510
Phone (202) 224-3121 (see below)

U.S. House of Representatives
Washington, DC 20515
Phone (202) 224-3121
(This is the Capitol Hill switchboard. Having
dialed this number, you can request the office of
any member of the House or Senate.)

Appendix A

American Life League

American Life League, the nation's largest Christian pro-life activist organization, concentrates its efforts on involving every American in the pro-life effort and helping them to use their talents in the area where they will be most comfortable. Here are a few examples of activities American Life League advocates that do stop abortion:

1. Counseling pregnant women, including giving them complete information on the status of their own pregnancy and at the same time the development of the child.

2. Sharing educational information with churches, civic organizations, student bodies, school boards and parent-teacher associations. There is an immense amount of colorful, positive pro-life educational material available that simply informs the average person of the real humanity of a child in the womb.

3. Lobbying legislators at the local, county, state and federal levels. By involving themselves in the political process, pro-life people can deliver three to five percent of the vote and make it very uncomfortable for politicians to continue to say that they are "personally opposed to abortion" while in fact they vote for abortion.

4. Picketing abortion clinics and referral agencies. Pro-life people are making a statement to the community that killing or promotion of it is going on within the buildings. This not only educates those who pass by but at the same time provokes members of the media to ask pointed questions about such demonstrations. In the end these demonstrations will be extremely effective. At the same time the picketing is going on, members of the pro-life community can also engage in peaceful sidewalk counseling, which is nothing more than giving total information abut the preborn baby to those women and men who have decided that they must for some reason kill an innocent human being.

Write me a letter and tell me what you would like to do to help save these innocent little babies created in the image and likeness of God, what you think you can accomplish in your own family, in your community, with members of your church or with the members of a civic organization to which you belong. American Life League will be able to help you do it just a little bit better than you thought you could.

Judie Brown
American Life League
P.O. Box 1350
Stafford, VA 22554

Appendix B

Love Is Out, Sin Is In!

The current efforts of "promosexual" groups like
Planned Parenthood Federation of America,
Center for Population Options, and others to place
a "clinic" in all junior and senior high schools are
causing great concern. America once had a public
education system dedicated to objective truth. It
now has chaos.

The "system" has opened its doors to public
health professionals and community leaders who,
"concerned" with the "epidemic" of teenage
pregnancy, actually believe that human sexuality is
merely a simple mechanical activity.

They discuss their own brand of "facts"
designed specifically to destroy the value system
which so thinly separates our way of life from that
of a barbaric society.

To them, sex is nothing more than a blind and
selfish instinct among beasts. And the beasts (which

you and I would identify as young children) need animal-trainers. The school-based sex clinic is simply the animal hospital.

If this sounds absurd to you, remember that Faye Wattleton, President of Planned Parenthood Federation of America, said on the McNeil-Lehrer program that, after all, there is birth control for roaches. Why not for teens?

What are the real facts?

● The **epidemic** is adolescent promiscuity, not adolescent pregnancy.

● The "1 million teenage pregnancies" you read about contain more than 650,000 pregnancies of young people who are married.

● The role of parents as primary educators of their children has been eroded to the point where most parents truly believe they are incapable of handling their own children in the area of human sexuality.

● The adolescent who uses the birth control pill has a one-in-eight chance of suffering from a dreaded pelvic inflammatory disease, a condition that can leave her sterile.

● The use of the birth control pill will not prevent AIDS.

● The condom is only 70 percent to 90 percent effective in preventing AIDS.

● School-based sex clinic studies themselves are fraught with error, leading the public to believe that teen pregnancies decrease where clinics are in use. However, the statistics provided by these clinics count a pregnancy only when a child is born. Babies slaughtered by abortion are not counted as pregnancies at all!

● The involvement of the federal government in permissive sex education (that is, how-to lessons in plumbing) has been a dismal failure. These programs began in 1965, from which time this nation has seen dramatic increases in adolescent pregnancy, adolescent abortion, adolescent venereal disease and adolescent depression.

● As early as 1968, studies of young people exposed to permissive sex education showed that it had liberalized student attitudes toward casual sex, homosexuality and pornography.

What is our response?

Human sexuality is a gift from God. But because God has been banned from the public education system, the word "sin" has been deleted from the vocabulary as well.

If I could say something to the millions of young people in our society who are presently victims of the co-opted public education system, I would simply repeat what was written in 1928 by

Rev. Daniel Lord:

"God—you see—when He placed upon mankind the terrible responsibility for human life, this participation in His power of creation, knew that He was fearfully burdening men and women.

"To bring children into the world, to assume the responsibility for their eternal destiny, to suffer as mothers have to suffer and to make the sacrifices that fathers have to make—well, it was asking a lot; and God never asks without giving abundantly in return.

"So into the hearts of men and women He poured this tremendous attraction and joy and exhiliration and sympathy and mutual impulse called love. It is something so beautiful that nobody has ever been able to really explain it.

"Men and women clasp hands and take up the burden of parenthood, not so much because they are aware of their cooperation with God in peopling the world and filling heaven as because they are drawn toward each other powerfully, delightfully, most irresistibly.

"A great desire to unite their lives, their futures, their thoughts, their bodies, flings them together in a happiness that is beyond any other purely natural happiness of earth. So God gives mankind in return for their participation in His divine creatorship the marvelous thing called love.

"Love is God's gift—God's way of drawing men and women toward each other; and it is His reward for their share in the creation of His little children."

Who will teach the lesson?

The school-based sex clinic will not teach this lesson, though. It cannot. Those who promote its existence fly in the face of love by promoting that sin which will rob our children of perhaps ever experiencing love.

You and I must teach this lesson.

● Do not permit the Governor's Task Force on Infant Mortality or the Governor's Task Force on Adolescent Pregnancy in your state to approve school-based sex clinics.

● Do not permit the March of Dimes and the American Red Cross to convince the parents of young people in your communtiy that school-based sex clinics are a "good idea."

● Start now to make your voice heard. It is your responsibility and mine as adults to lead the way. The hour is late.

By (Mrs.) Judie Brown. This appendix first appeared as a column in Liberty Report, *February, 1987.*

Notes

(Including a bibliography of worthwhile reading)

1 *How Babies Grow* (Stafford VA: American
   Life League, 1984); brochure; ALL no. AB2.
2 *The Dangers of the Pill and the IUD*
   (Stafford VA: American Life League, 1984);
   packet, ALL no. NF2.
3 Robert G. Marshall & Herbert Ratner, MD,
   *'Oral Contraceptives': The Medical Evidence
   for Covert Abortion* (Stafford VA: American
   Life League, 1986); reprint.
4 Gary Bergel, *Abortion in America*
   (Reston VA: Intercessors for America, 1980);
   pamphlet.
5 Bernard N. Nathanson, MD, *The Abortion
   Papers: Inside the Abortion Mentality*
   (New York: Frederick Fell Publishers, 1983).
6 Robert G. Marshall, *The Big Lie: The Extent*

of Illegal Abortion (Stafford VA: American Life League, 1985); pamphlet, ALL no. AB24.

7 Ann Saltenberger, *Every Woman Has a Right to Know the Dangers of Legal Abortion* (Glassboro NJ: Air Plus Industries, 1975).

8 Robert G. Marshall, *The Collapse of American Justice* (Stafford VA: American Life League, 1984); booklet, ALL no. BO13.

9 Robert G. Marshall, *Is Abortion Safer Than Childbirth? Reasons for Doubt* (Stafford VA: American Life League, 1984); pamphlet, ALL no. AB6.

10 Anne Speckhard, *Psychological Aspects of Stress Following Abortion* (Arlington VA: Family Assistance Center, 1986).

11 David Mall & Walter F. Watts, MD, eds., *The Psychological Aspects of Abortion,* (Washington DC: University Publications of America, 1979).

12 A directory of post-abortion counselng services is available from American Life League, PO Box 1350, Stafford VA 22554. The organizations offering these services are also listed in the white and/or yellow pages of the telephone directory.

13 Elasah Drogin, *Margaret Sanger: Father of Modern Society* (Catholics United for Life Press, 1986).

14 Julian Simon, *The Ultimate Resource*
    (Princeton NJ: Princeton Univ. Press, 1981).
15 John F. Kippley, *Birth Control and Christian
    Discipline* (Cincinnati OH: Couple to Couple
    League International, Inc., 1985); pamphlet.
16 Daniel Overduin, PhD, & John I. Fleming,
    Life in a Test-Tube (Adelaide, Australia:
    Lutheran Publishing House, 1982); book,
    ALL no. EG6.
17 Planned Parenthood Federation of America,
    1985 Annual Service Report (New York).
18 Murray Norris, PhD, JD, *Weep for Your
    Children* (Clovis CA: Christian Family
    Renewal, 1975); booklet, ALL no. SH2.
19 Prof. Charles Rice, *The Human Life
    Amendment: An Introduction* (Stafford VA:
    American Life League, 1986); brochure, ALL
    no. AB1.
20 Congressman Thomas J. Bliley (VA),
    *Rape and Incest Exception Not Needed and
    Unwarranted* (Stafford VA: American Life
    League); reprinted from the Congressional
    Record for July 25, 1983; ALL no. AB22.
21 A good one is the *Pro-Life Media Handbook*
    by Judie Brown (Stafford VA: Anastasia
    Books, 1980); ALL no. BO2.

Index

A

aborted babies
    burial of bodies — 18
    disposal of bodies — 18, 58
abortion — 129
    and big business — 67
    and "defective" children — 91
    as a business — 17
    as a social issue — 105
    birth control pill — 13
    complications from — 25-31
    cost — 17
    during the ninth month — 19
    economics of — 77
    IUD — 13
    outlawing — 19-20
    RU 486 — 14
    safety — 32, 97, 123

surgical methods	15, 16
when most are performed	16
abortion clinic	17, 58, 59
franchises	66
practices	61
Adams, John	87, 107
AIDS	123, 129, 131
Alan Guttmacher Institute	131
ALLPAC	140, 144
Allred, Dr.	67
alternate lifestyles	132
amniocentesis	124
Anglican Church	42
animal, man as	7, 48
anti-abortion movement	7
assisted suicide	73, 78

B

Baby Jane Doe	117
Bible	
and pregnancy (John 16:21)	33
Book of Jeremiah	5
creation	5, 6
solutions	108
Bill of Rights	55
birth control	11
and churches	42, 43
and teenagers	77, 95, 122,

                                          123, 133
birth control pill   12, 13, 56
Birthright   34
Brown, Louise   46

                    C
caesarean section abortion   16
cancer of the uterus (womb)   112
capital punishment   125
chastity   121, 122, 131
chemical abortion   14, 16
child abuse   83, 84, 97
China and abortion   39
"choice"   81, 82, 95
chorionic villus biopsy   124
Civil War   106
compromise
    and church leaders   42-44, 79, 104
    and pro-life groups   153-156
Comstock Laws   54
conception   2
conservative   48
Constitution   54, 55,
                                          87, 155
contraception   11, 12

                    D
Declaration of Independence   6

"death with dignity"   90, 97
"defective" children   91
Democrats   154, 157
Dewey, John   44
dilatation and curretage   15
Down's Syndrome   117
Dred Scott decision   93

                         E
elderly   8, 71-78, 118
      financial drain?   73, 77
environmental groups   48
Equal Rights Amendment   64
Ehrlich, Paul   41
Espinosa, M.D., Jose   25
Ethiopia   134
eugenics   38
euthanasia   71-75, 129,
                                           130
"every child a wanted child"   96
Exit   72

                         F
Feminist Women's Health Center   66
fertilization   2, 86
fetal development   2-4, 92
fetus   92, 95
Ford Foundation   42, 68

Friedan, Betty   45

G
General Motors   42
gun control   127
Guttmacher, M.D., Alan   40

H
handicapped newborn infants   8, 116-118,
                                 124, 126
    parents of   120
Hemlock Society   72
Hitler, Adolf   38
homosexuality   132, 133
How Babies Grow   2
Humanist Manifesto   102
human life amendment   142, 143
Humphry, Derek   72, 78
hypernatremic abortion   15, 16
hysterotomy abortion   16

I
IBM   68
illegal abortion
    and doctors   21
    and women   20, 21
    deaths from   23
    "imposing a religious belief"   86, 97

implantation	2, 13
incest	115, 116
International Planned Parenthood	
Federation	134
in vitro fertilization	46, 47, 86
IRS and the church	100
IUD (intrauterine device)	13, 56

J

Jewish pro-life effort	105

K

"keep legislators out of my	
bedroom"	87, 88, 97
Kellogg Corporation	68

L

Lambeth Conference	42
Landers, Ann	121
legal starvation	74, 75
"legislating morality"	86, 87, 97,
	154, 155
lesbianism	132
letter to the editor	147, 148
liability and parental rights	60, 61
liberal	48
living will	8, 79, 90, 91,
	97

M

Malthus, Thomas	40
March of Dimes	65, 66
man as animal	7, 48
media influences	132
mentality of death	
defined	71
in practice	76, 77, 83, 84, 120, 130, 134, 135
Michael Fund	66
Moore, Hugh	41, 134

N

National Organization for Women	63, 64, 82
"New Right"	153, 154
nuclear war	124, 125

P

parental rights	52, 53, 57-62, 95
pastors and politics	149
peace movement	124, 125
PG-13	132
placenta	15
Planned Parenthood	
corporate support for	68, 69
counseling	25

founder of	37
income from abortion	65
philosophy of	38, 39, 84, 95, 113, 114, 121, 122
politicians and	150, 151
sex instruction	132-133
political action	139-146
political labels	49
politicians, defined	154, 155
population control	39, 40
and government support	42
pornography	132, 133
"potential" human being	1
Potomac Fever	155
poverty	126
press conference	146-147
press, working with	144-148
"product of conception"	92, 93, 95
pro-life movement	7, 8
promiscuity	121, 122, 131, 133
prostaglandin abortion	16
Protestants and pro-life	105, 106

Q

"quality of life"	88, 89, 91, 96, 117

R

racism   38
    and Margaret Sanger   38
rape   112-115
Ratner, M.D., Herbert   25
"reproductive freedom"   89
Republican   48, 157
right to life movement   7
right to privacy   44, 87, 88, 96
    and the Supreme Court   54, 55
Rockefeller   42, 68
Roman Catholic Church
    and population control   41
    and pro-life movement   105
RU 486   12, 14, 15

S

saline abortion   15
Saltenberger, Ann   25
Sanger, Margaret   37, 38, 41, 44
"save the life of the mother"   111-112
school-based clinics   60, 131,
                                          163-167
secular humanism   6
"separation of church and state"   100-102
"sexual freedom"   89, 96, 122
sex education, basic   130
sex instruction   129-133

shepherding homes   119
sin   43, 108, 109
Slee, Noah   41
Speckhard, Ph.D., Anne   33
spina bifida   117, 118
"squeal rule"   94, 95
starvation, legalized   74, 75, 117
Steinem, Gloria   45
sterilization   134
suction abortion   15
Supreme Court and:
    abortion   45, 51-53,
                                55-59
    Dred Scott, 1857   93, 94
    hospitalizaton before abortion   58
    humane treatment of aborted
        babies   58
    informed consent   31, 32, 58-60
    parental rights   52, 53, 58-62
    paternal (father's) rights   53
    secular humanism as religion   102
    waiting period before abortion   59
Supreme Court decisions
    City of Akron v. Akron
        Center for Reproductive
        Health   57-60
    Eisenstadt v. Baird   55
    Griswold v. Connecticut   54

Planned Parenthood v.
    Danforth   52, 53
Roe v. Wade, Doe v. Bolton   51, 94
Torcaso v. Watkins   102

T

teenage pregnancy   121-123, 131
teenage promiscuity   122, 123
terminal illness   75
    treatment for   75, 76
Three-In-One Oil   41, 42
tubal pregnancy   111

U

unemancipated minor   52, 53
United Nations Fund for Popula-
    tion Activities (UNFPA)   134
U.S. Government
    church and state   100-102
    funding abortion   17, 35, 42,
                                           132, 133
    funding population control 42
    regulations to protect han-
        dicapped newborn infants 118
United Way   66
unity   105-110,
                                           124-127
"unwanted"   83-85, 96

Upjohn Pharmaceutical Company   16

V

Van Buren, Abigail   121
venereal disease   122, 129-131

W

Washington, George   87, 107
"womb as war zone"   85, 125
women
    "right to control own body"   85, 96
    more than one abortion   17
    who seek abortion   19
women's rights groups   32, 34

Z

Zero Population Growth   64, 65
zygote   13, 92